FAT SEX: NEW DIRECTIONS IN THEORY AND ACTIVISM

Gender, Bodies and Transformation

Series editor: Meredith Jones,
University of Technology, Sydney, Australia

This series explores the intersection of two key themes in relation to scholarship on bodies: gender and transformation. Bodies are gendered via biology, culture, medicine and society, such that gender, so deeply and intimately connected to identity, is a crucial part of any thorough analysis of the body. At the same time, bodies are – and have always been – sites of transformation, whether through 'natural' processes such as pregnancy, illness and ageing, or the more eye-catching, 'unnatural' transformations of cosmetic surgery, violence, extreme bodybuilding or dieting, cross-species transplantation, elective amputation or tattooing.

Interdisciplinary in scope and welcoming work from a range of approaches, including cultural and media studies, sociology, gender studies, feminist theory, phenomenology, queer studies and ethnography, *Gender, Bodies and Transformation* publishes scholarly examinations of contemporary cultural changes that are relevant to both gender and the transformation of bodies, whether in single bodies or between bodies.

Also in the series

Sport, Gender and Power
The Rise of Roller Derby
Adele Pavlidis and Simone Fullagar

The Weight of Images
Affect, Body Image and Fat in the Media
Katariina Kyrölä

Fat Sex: New Directions in Theory and Activism

Edited by

HELEN HESTER
Middlesex University, UK

CAROLINE WALTERS
BiUK

Routledge
Taylor & Francis Group
LONDON AND NEW YORK

First published 2015 by Ashgate Publishing

2 Park Square, Milton Park, Abingdon, Oxfordshire OX14 4RN
52 Vanderbilt Avenue, New York, NY 10017

Routledge is an imprint of the Taylor & Francis Group, an informa business

First issued in paperback 2020

British Library Cataloguing in Publication Data
A catalogue record for this book is available from the British Library.

The Library of Congress has cataloged the printed edition as follows:
Fat sex : new directions in theory and activism / [edited by] Helen Hester and Caroline Walters.
pages cm. -- (Gender, bodies and transformation)
Includes bibliographical references and index.
ISBN 978-1-4724-3254-4 (hardback)
1. Sex. 2. Overweight persons--Sexual behavior. 3. Pornography in popular culture.
I. Hester, Helen, 1983- editor. II. Walters, Caroline, editor.

HQ23.F38 2015
306.7--dc23

2014048304

ISBN 978-1-4724-3254-4 (hbk)
ISBN 978-0-367-59887-7 (pbk)

Contents

CREATIVE INTERLUDE

THE PORNOGRAPHY OF FAT

CREATIVE INTERLUDE

CULTURALLY (IN)VISIBLE BODIES

CREATIVE INTERLUDE

About the Editors

Helen Hester is Lecturer in Promotional Cultures at Middlesex University, London. Her research interests include technofeminism, sexuality studies and theories of embodiment, and she is a member of the international feminist collective Laboria Cuboniks. She is the author of *Beyond Explicit: Pornography and the Displacement of Sex* (SUNY Press, 2014), the co-editor of the collection *Dea ex Machina* (Merve, 2015), and the series editor for Ashgate's 'Sexualities in Society' book series.

Caroline Walters is a research associate for BiUK (The UK Organisation for Research on Bisexuality). Her research interests include fat studies, sexuality studies and mental health. She is working on a book on gender, BDSM and culture.

Notes on Contributors

Vikki Chalklin is a queer fat femme performer, activist and scholar based in London. Her research interests are primarily located at the intersection of queer theory, body theory and visual culture and performance studies, investigating what considerations of affect, relationality and embodied subjectivity can bring to the study of art, performance and queer cultural production. Alongside teaching and academic research, her performance practice works to blur the boundaries between her creative and scholarly worlds, giving cabaret-style performances of academic work at conferences, and performance lectures at queer performance and cabaret clubs. New projects currently in development examine fat activism and performance, the relationship between queer and feminist pornography and histories of performance and body art, and the resistant possibilities of contemporary dance practice.

Kimberly Dark is a writer, mother, performer and professor. She is the author of five award-winning solo performance scripts and her poetry and prose appear in a number of publications. She teaches in a graduate program in Sociological Practice at Cal State San Marcos and tours widely in North America, Europe and Australia.

Kimberly's work engages audiences with surprising topics. Using humour and intimacy she reveals the contours of privilege and oppression in our daily lives. The *Salt Lake Tribune* in Utah says 'Dark doesn't shy away from provocative, incendiary statements, but don't expect a rant. Her shows, leavened with humor, are more likely to explore how small everyday moments can inform the arc of our lives'. The *High Plains Reader* in Fargo, North Dakota says 'Dark's skill as a storyteller gets to your heart by exposing hers'.

Jeannine A. Gailey is Associate Professor of Sociology in the Department of Sociology and Anthropology at Texas Christian University. Her research and teaching interests include: sociology of the body, fat studies, gender and sexuality, deviance, and organisational wrongdoing. She is the author of the book *The Hyper(in)visible Fat Woman: Weight and Gender Discourse in Contemporary Society*. Additionally, her work has appeared in journals such as *Social Psychology Quarterly, Fat Studies Journal, Deviant Behavior, Critical Criminology, Qualitative Research,* and *Journal of Gender Studies.*

Michelle Green is a postgraduate student in the department of American and Canadian Studies at the University of Nottingham. Her thesis examines othering, trauma and the pursuit of selfhood in representations of fatness and 'obesity' in contemporary U.S. fiction. Michelle's wider interests include medical moral panics, gender and genre theory, and contemporary Anglo-American writing.

Frances Hatherley is a doctoral candidate in Art and Design at Middlesex University. Her research examines the potential for a radical working-class aesthetics in formations of grotesque and sublime femininities in visual culture. She also writes on British politics, body and dress, space and education. She has a chapter published in the book *Everyday Surrealism* (Edition Text und Kritik, 2012) exploring rebellious female grotesques in *The Hearing Trumpet* and *Grey Gardens*. She also runs a blog *The Red Deeps* where discussions of class and education run alongside sexuality, art, literature and popular culture.

Natalie Ingraham, MPH is a PhD candidate in Sociology at the University of California, San Francisco. She is also a Research Project Coordinator at Lyon-Martin Health Services in San Francisco. Her dissertation work and research interests focus on intersections between body size, gender, sexuality and health. Ingraham received a BS in Psychology from the University of Science and Arts of Oklahoma and a Master's Degree in Public Health from Indiana University, Bloomington. Her work on queer pornography has also been featured in the *International Journal of Multiple Research Approaches* and additional work in critical obesity/fat studies has been featured in *Women's Health Issues* and *Fat Studies*.

Laura Ellen Joyce lectures in film and literature at Edinburgh Napier University. She was project co-ordinator of the AHRC Global Queer Cinema network between 2012–2013. Her first novel, *The Museum of Atheism*, was published in November 2012 by Salt. Her second novel, *The Luminol Reels*, was published by Calamari Archive in August 2014.

Goda Klumbyte has recently earned a Research MA degree in Media Studies at Utrecht University. She has presented at conferences including: 'NOG National Research Day' (University of Nijmegen, 2012) and 'Thinking on the Edge of Cuts: Inspirations and Innovations in Gender Studies' (University of Leeds, 2011). She tutored at the NOISE Gender Studies Summer School in 2012. Her academic interests include pornography studies, feminist media and technology studies, and critical theory. She is also a co-editor of a Lithuanian online feminist magazine 'Digėlė'. Her essay 'Wired Fingers, Sticky Keyboards: Towards an Embodied Approach to Internet Pornography' is included in *Everyday Feminist Research Praxis: Doing Gender in the Netherlands* (Cambridge Scholars, 2014; eds. with Domitilla Olivieri and Koen Leurs).

Jennifer Lee is Lecturer in Creative Writing, Literary Studies and Gender Studies at Victoria University in Melbourne, Australia. She researches in the interdisciplinary fields of Fat Studies and Creative Writing (often producing work that crosses into both disciplines). During her PhD she researched the treatment of intersex bodies in Western culture in order to write a novel.

Jennifer has published and presented at conferences in Australia, New Zealand, the US, the UK, Spain, Portugal and Italy. She is currently co-editing a creative anthology, *Fat Mook* (part magazine, part book), with another Australian Fat Studies scholar, Jackie Wykes. Jennifer has a long history of curating queer events for Midsumma Festival, the queer arts and culture festival in Melbourne. Her last sold-out event for Midsumma was 'Dangerous Curves Ahead' – eight performers exploring intersections of fat and queer. She is currently focused on writing memoir, narrative non-fiction and autoethnographic work about the fat body. Her most recently published short stories include characters that are transgendered superheroes and genetically-altered bisexual spies and can be read in the US queer genre collection *Clones, Fairies and Monsters in the Closet* (Lee, 2013).

Sarah Parker is Impact Research Fellow at the University of Stirling. She recently published her first monograph, *The Lesbian Muse and Poetic Identity, 1889–1930* (Pickering & Chatto, 2013). Her other publications include 'Fashioning Michael Field: Michael Field and Late-Victorian Dress Culture' (*Journal of Victorian Culture*, 2013), 'Whose Muse? Sappho, Swinburne and Amy Lowell' in *Algernon Charles Swinburne: Unofficial Laureate* (Manchester UP, 2013) and '"A Girl's Love": Lord Alfred Douglas as Homoerotic Muse in the Poetry of Olive Custance' (*Women: A Cultural Review*, 2011). She is currently working on her second monograph, entitled 'Women Poets, Self-Fashioning and Photography at the Fin de Siècle (1880–1914)'.

Cat Pausé (@FOMNZ) is a Fat Studies Researcher and Lecturer in Human Development at Massey University, New Zealand. Her research focuses on the construction, revision, and maintenance of spoiled identities and its effects on health and well-being of fat individuals. She is a co-editor of *Queering Fat Embodiment* (Ashgate, 2014), and has published in *Feminist Review*, *Somatechnics*, and *Narrative Inquiries in Bioethics*. Cat hosted the 'Fat Studies: Reflective Intersections' conference in New Zealand (2012), and guest edited an issue on intersectionality for *Fat Studies: An Interdisciplinary Journal of Body Weight and Society*. Her work has been featured in *The Huffington Post*, Yahoo, NPR, Radio New Zealand, the *Daily Mail*, and 20/20. Cat engages in the fatosphere through her blog, Tumblr, and podcast, Friend of Marilyn.

Zora Simic is a lecturer in history and convenor of Women's and Gender Studies at the University of New South Wales, Sydney, Australia. She researches the past and present of western feminisms and has published widely in these areas, in specialised journals and for mainstream publications. With Monica Dux, she is the co-author of *The Great Feminist Denial* (Melbourne University Press, 2008), an examination of popular debates about feminism.

Katrine Smiet is a PhD candidate in feminist philosophy at Radboud University Nijmegen, Netherlands. Her research interests include theories of embodiment, feminist phenomenology, critical race theory and intersectionality. She is active in the Utrecht-based feminist group Feministisch Verzet.

Alison Winch is a poet and critic. Her monograph, *Girlfriends and Postfeminist Sisterhood* (Palgrave, 2014) examines how neoliberal branded cultures penetrate intimate female networks. Her poems have been published in *Rialto*, and *Magma*, among others. She is currently working on her first collection.

Acknowledgements

We are indebted to the team at Ashgate Publishing, particularly Neil Jordan, who has believed in this project from the very beginning. His encouragement and expert guidance throughout the publication process has been extremely helpful and very much appreciated.

Helen Hester

I would like to thank my co-editor, Caroline Walters, for making the process of assembling this volume such a pleasure. Thanks are also due to Diarmuid Hester, Lisa Darms, Sarah Taylor-Harman, Alex Dymock, Michael O'Rourke, Feona Attwood, and Merja Makinen for their invaluable advice, and to Nick Srnicek for his on-going support and seemingly inexhaustible patience. Finally, I want to thank all the authors who have contributed to this collection; it has been a real pleasure to work with such a wonderful assortment of activists and scholars.

Caroline Walters

I would like to thank my co-editor, Helen Hester, for making this process enjoyable and providing encouragement and support throughout. I want to thank Kirsty Fife for introducing me to fat activism and fat studies back in 2007, as without her this project would never have existed. Extra thanks go to Jude Roberts, Meg John Barker, Jessica Worden, Feona Attwood, Hannele Harjunen, my friends at Irreverent Dance, and my family for their support and advice along the way. Special thanks go to Adrian Scoffield, who has been gentle, kind and patient with me throughout the process but especially during the final months. Finally, I also want to thank all of the authors who have contributed to this collection and helping make our vision for a book on fat sex a reality; it has been a pleasure to work with and encourage your wonderful ideas.

Chapter 1

Riots Not Diets!: Sex, Fat Studies and DIY Activism

Helen Hester and Caroline Walters

Fat Sex and its Academic Absence

Fat studies, which has roots in fat activism, emerges as a response to a contemporary cultural landscape that is openly hostile towards fat people and their perceived social and aesthetic transgressions. This book builds on a deep admiration for this discipline and examines the relationship between fat, sex and sexuality. It follows in the wake of key texts – including *The Fat Studies Reader* (eds. Rothblum and Solovay, 2009), Deborah Lupton's *Fat* (2012), and the academic journal *Fat Studies: An Interdisciplinary Journal of Body Weight and Society* – which have broken new ground in the debates around fat embodiment. Their insights encompass issues such as health and the medicalization of 'body mass', cultural geographies of weight and size, and fatness and social justice. The discipline has been ahead of the curve, too, in understanding how intersecting forms of oppression impact embodiment. It has consistently demonstrated a commitment to better understanding the ways in which factors such as class, gender, race, age, ability, ethnicity, and sexuality can inform one another and shape the lived realities of fat people. *Fat Sex: New Directions in Theory and Activism* owes a debt to this activism infused scholarship, and seeks to draw on the strengths of the tradition in order to make a contribution to the field.

But while fat studies as an emerging discipline demonstrates an extraordinary sensitivity to issues that have frequently been neglected within other forms of scholarly debate, there appears to be a gap within the literature when it comes to theorizing fat sex. While there have been one or two important and insightful essays on the topic (Murray 2004, Gailey and Prohaska 2006), it is only with very recent additions to the field, such as *Queering Fat Embodiment* (Pausé, Wykes and Murray, 2014), that the insights of fat studies and sexuality studies have been brought together. There is much more that might be done to facilitate a sustained and productive conversation between these traditions, and to help further detailed critical engagement around the intersection of size and sex. Contributions from diverse perspectives are certainly to be encouraged, and this volume is an attempt to foster such diversity. *Fat Sex: New Directions in Theory and*

Activism aims to address the lack of dedicated scholarship, and is one of the first academic texts to focus exclusively and directly on fat sex.

Fat (and) Sex: Activist and Community Origins

Although academic material on fat sex has been slow to emerge, there is a richer and more respected tradition of writing on this topic to be found within the sphere of activism, self-help, and (auto)biography. Hanne Blank's *Big Big Love: A Sex and Relationships Guide for People of Size* (2011) and Rebecca Jane Weinstein's *Fat Sex: The Naked Truth* (2012), for example, provide different (though similarly sex- and fat-positive) perspectives on fat embodiment, and seek to reflect on the specificities of sexual practices, intimacies, and relationships for 'people of size'. Works specifically dedicated to fat sex are complemented by texts that include issues of sex and sexuality as part of broader discussions about fat life experiences. Virgie Tovar's collection *Hot and Heavy: Fierce Fat Girls on Life, Love, and Fashion* (2012) would be one example here, drawing as it does from a range of voices to offer short reflections on the topics of sex, identity and the fat female form. These are accessibly written texts, aimed at delivering a body-positive message to a broad general audience. As reflected by Weinstein's text, whose publication was crowd-funded via a Kickstarter campaign, there is often a spirited and enterprising DIY ethos to be found behind much of this literature, and indeed, behind fat sex activism more generally.

In some cases, this ethos is explicitly linked to the radical amateurism of counter-cultural movements such as punk and riot grrrl, which have distinctive traditions of self-publishing. Within the Tammy Rae Carland Zine Collection (located within New York University's Riot Grrrl Archive), one can find numerous examples of fat activism within the feminist zine cultures of the 1990s. In some cases, this manifests itself as individual articles within general interest zines; *Everybody Sucks But Me*, for example, subversively vandalizes found material on the topic of 'Fat and How Not to Be' (n.d.), while queer punk fanzine *Three Dollar Bill* seeks to raise awareness about the systematic oppression of fat people, and to encourage closer ties between fat liberation and lesbian feminist movements ('Fat Oppression and Fat Liberation', 1991). In other cases, activism takes the form of publications specifically dedicated to exploring issues of fat embodiment from a riot grrrl perspective – *The Adventures of Big Girl* (1993), for example, or *I'm So Fucking Beautiful* (n.d.).

These publications address a range of issues, from clothes shopping and street harassment to diet culture and self-acceptance, but what is important for our purposes is their tendency to include sex (and sexual pleasure) as an integral part of their diverse political projects. *I'm So Fucking Beautiful* (n.d.), for example, discusses the author's embodied experiences of the sensuality of fat flesh ('fat is fun! […] fun to suck on'), and accompanies many of its articles with erotically-tinged nude sketches of fat female bodies. *The Nerdy Grrrl Revolution* (n.d.), meanwhile, includes a personal reflection on the difficulty of being desired for one's fatness – an experience that is problematized for the author after she receives sexually explicitly fan mail. Within this riot grrrl tradition, then, sex – whether painful, problematic, or pleasurable – is shown to play an important role in fat embodiment.

Inspired by the punk movement and DIY culture was one of the most influential fat activist zines: *FaT GiRL: A Zine for Fat Dykes and the Women Who Want Them*, which ran from 1994 until 1997. It was compiled and published by the FaT GiRL Collective based in San Francisco, but had international contributors, featuring work by Charlotte Cooper, Sondra Solovay, Max Airborne and Judy Freespirit. It was an expansive zine, with each issue coming in at 60 pages of A4, and included stories, interviews, comics, poetry and an incredible array of photo spreads showing fat women enjoying sex. The collective members wanted to present a diverse array of fat lesbian bodies and to challenge cultural norms of appropriateness. Its ever-present politics, explicit sexual representations and size meant that this was one of the few fat zines that academics have written about (Snider 2009). In chapters 2 and 3 of this book, Zora Simic and Cat Pausé respectively, consider this zine's legacy, its position within fat activism, and its contribution to representing fat queer sexuality.

The people who produce these zines – many of whom present themselves as young, female, queer, and/or economically disempowered – do the work of consciousness-raising within their own communities, while also sharing experiences, coping strategies, and subcultural knowledge about fat sex. The publication of contact details and the culture of non-monetary exchange (in which the price of a zine is often advertised as a simple zine for zine swap) enable these writers to engage in semi-anonymized conversations. This facilitates unique ways of building networks, obtaining support, and enabling knowledge exchange around culturally-loaded issues. The self-publishing tradition also gives fat punks the space to run against the received wisdom about sex, size, and their intersection. Zinesters write fat sexual practices and the fat sexual body *against* those mainstream knowledges that typically exclude and produce them. In this sense, we can position queer punk and riot grrrl zine making as part of a culture of determined and resistant amateurism. It resists hegemonic understandings about fat sex by clearing a subcultural space for certain marginalized voices.

We can see the legacy of this DIY culture in numerous strands of fat activism today. Hard copy zine making continues to have its place and many activists use it as a tool in their practice, but we can also see the continuance of the self-publishing tradition in a different form in the wake of the development of Web 2.0. As the use of personal blogs and social networking sites has become increasingly common, activists have sought to exploit these platforms in order to agitate for fat liberation and to build communities. In recent years a number of tumblrs have emerged seeking to challenge preconceptions about the politics of size and sex; fat-sex-is-good-sex.tumblr.com (n.d.), fat-sex.tumblr.com (n.d.), and fatsexadvice.tumblr.com (n.d.), for example, are all dedicated to the topic. Microblogs of this kind tend to incorporate a mixture of practical advice, comical memes, and sexually explicit imagery of various kinds as part of a multi-faceted engagement with fat sex. The repurposing and re-contextualizing of existing material that takes place through 'reblogging', as well as the prevalence of user-generated content, strongly recalls certain elements of 90s zine culture.

These sites retain an interest in the kind of sex- and body-positive messaging demonstrated by riot grrrl publications, and continue to avow a commitment to providing resources for their communities: 'Here we believe that good sex is not dependant on your weight. Need some advice? Ask away. Tired of not seeing your body type represented in porn? We will find it' (fatsexadvice.tumblr.com, n.d.). While we might seek to problematize uncritical assumptions about the value of activism based on locating and sharing pornographic images of particular body types, there is no denying that these virtual materials speak in some way to the politics of fat sex. A particular version of what fat sex is and means is generated by these tumblrs, and they make accessible a particular form of visibility for big bodies – one which courts an overt recognition of their sexuality. Indeed, the potential role of pornographic imagery in twenty-first century fat activism is an issue that needs to be addressed, and is discussed by several of the authors included in this volume (see Ingraham, Smiet and Klumbyte). This attention to porn, and to the labour that produces it, is arguably one of the unique strengths of this text.

Despite the lack of relevant scholarly research there are a number of extremely rich and interesting traditions dealing with the topic of size and sex to be found elsewhere. This is something that *Fat Sex: New Directions in Theory and Activism* is keen to acknowledge, and the collection is influenced by (and engages with) some of the innovative work being done by artists, activists, and para-academics. This book seeks to demonstrate some of the ways in which academics are also activists and activists are also academics, since the boundaries between these two seemingly commonsensical categories are often less clear-cut than they might appear. For example, many of the contributors to this collection straddle the boundary between academia and activism. Several activists have contributed to the volume, and their strategies for raising awareness, challenging preconceptions, and advocating for a culturally stigmatized community inform much of the material included here. At the same time, however, various strategies of 'making visible' are critiqued and challenged, as the way forward for political agitation and cultural representation is debated. The result is a cutting-edge exploration not only of fat sex, but also of identity politics and contemporary body activism in general. This collection will seek to build on the important contributions of the activist community, bringing debates about fat sex into the academic arena, and providing a critical space for voices from across the spectrum of contemporary theory and activism.

Fat Sex: New Directions in Theory and Activism

While activism has long been influential in exploring fat sex, this is the first collection of work focused specifically on its critical and political potential. The chapters collected here cover a range of approaches to fat sex which draw from the traditions of history, sociology, performance studies, literary studies and gender studies. We hope that reading work from these different disciplines side by side will help to give the reader a more comprehensive picture of the interdisciplinary intellectual debates surrounding fat studies in general and, more specifically, fat sex. *Fat Sex* aims to be international as well as interdisciplinary, and the collection goes some way towards addressing Charlotte Cooper's concern that fat studies should really be called 'Fat American Studies' (2009, 327–333). Not only is the collection edited by two British academics, but it includes contributions from the UK, mainland Europe, the US, and Australasia. We hope that future work in this area will be able to further increase its global reach.

To help the reader traverse the complex material in this book we have arranged it in sections, beginning with general wide ranging debates before moving on to specific intersections between fat, sex and its representations. We outline the themes in these sections by explaining the function of each section and each chapter's contribution. While there are four categories, the material does overlap and speak to chapters in other sections, for the individual pieces are less discrete than the organiziation of this text may make them appear. The sections are: Fat Histories, Fat Communities; Fat Gender Politics; The Pornography of Fat; and Culturally (In)Visible Bodies.

Fat Histories, Fat Communities

In order to look forwards and forge new directions in research, we wanted the book to open by looking back at the histories of fat activists, academics, and writers who made the existence of this collection possible. With the advent of the fatosphere, it can be easy for many to think this phenomenon of being critical about fat is a new-fangled fad that arose in the wake of the obesity epidemic, which would be denying our histories. These chapters by Zora Simic and Cat Pausé explore the roots of contemporary considerations of fat sex by paying close attention to the complex legacies of fat activisms and early influential writings.

Zora Simic's chapter 'Fat as a Feminist Issue: A History' opens this book by tackling the legacies of fat feminisms and activisms, and by considering the ways in which feminisms have dealt with fat. This complex chapter helps to ground contemporary work on fat sex by providing the necessary contextual material. Its first section focuses on the development of fat feminism from the 1970s American pioneer fat activist group, Fat Underground, via the queer fat activism of the FaT GiRL collective in the 1990s, through to the fatosphere of the 2000s. The second part of her chapter examines mainstream critiques of fat by positioning two best-selling texts in their social and historical context: Susie Orbach's *Fat is a Feminist Issue* (1978) and Naomi Wolf's *The Beauty Myth* (1991). Simic's chapter provides readers with a useful foundation to the subsequent debates and discussions about fat sex by looking at the ways that a variety of previous writers and movements have dealt with these issues.

While Simic's chapter offers a historical overview, Cat Pausé's chapter focuses on work from the past decade and on the ways that representations of fat sex engage with prevalent anti-fat attitudes and discourses. Pausé reflects on why it is not surprising that fat sex is rarely discussed if the majority of empirical academic research focuses on reasons that people would be unhappy with their bodies, their size, and its negative impact on their sexual functioning. The second half of this chapter entitled 'Human Nature: On Fat Sexual Identity and Agency' considers a variety of activist books, websites and interventions that offer practical strategies and support for fat people to re-engage with their bodies and sexuality. Together these two chapters help to frame the focus of the book by positioning the academic research firmly within the tradition of fat studies, its relationship with feminisms and activism.

Fat Gender Politics

Since much of fat studies is written by women due to its roots within feminism (see Pausé, Chapter 2) it is unsurprising that several chapters in this book explicitly consider the ways in which gender, fat and sex intersect. This section serves to demarcate those chapters where gender and its political relationship with fat is a primary focus.

Chapter 4 by Jeannine Gailey entitled 'Transforming the Looking-Glass: Fat Women's Sexual Empowerment through Body Acceptance' is based on in-depth interviews with 74 North American fat women who talked with her about their sexual and dating experiences. Through this data Gailey discovers that embracing one's size can enable sexual empowerment and satisfaction. She considers the role of age, alternative sexual lifestyles (e.g. non-monogamy and BDSM), discovery of the fatosphere and online dating. This chapter contains many extensive quotations from Gailey's participants, which enables readers to follow her conclusions and disrupts the power dynamics between researcher and participant.

Frances Hatherley's chapter 'Against "Good Taste": Class, Corpulence and the Subversive Pleasures of "Unfit" Femininities' uses an intersectional approach to consider how class, fat and femininity become differently marked. She chooses not to use the word fat in this piece but rather corpulence, because for her 'it describes a body that is an overabundance, of almost pure corporeality. Its very bodiliness strongly connects it to the lower stratum, of the vulgar and the base. Likewise, the working class body shares many of these cultural associations with lowness and dirt'. This provides Hatherley with a framework for her intersectional analysis of ways that working class femininities can flout conceptions of good taste. In order to make this argument she uses the work of Bev Skeggs and Owen Jones to analyse how – at least in the UK – it is the middle-classes,who determine what is in 'good taste'.

Hatherley argues that the working class body has shifted from one of 'hard-working respectability to a *body* that is hated, despised and ridiculed: a body on which is written a brash, distasteful, lazy ignorance, a body seen as physically and socially "unfit"'. She argues this is particularly true of the fat female working class body. Using these conceptual ideas concerning feminine norms, Hatherley analyses enjoyment while looking at texts that represent these unruly bodies. She focuses on *The Fat Slags* comic strip by Graham Dury from 1989 and the enormous paintings of fleshy women by Jenny Saville. This chapter provides a valuable addition to the book for its explicit consideration of the relationship between fat, gender and class.

In 'All Hail the Fierce Fat Femmes', Vikki Chalklin takes readers to the world of London-based performance artist Scottee and the event *Hamburger Queen* that ran from 2011 to 2014. It was a 'beauty pageant and talent show for fat people' (Scottee 2014), where self-identified fat people could perform to become queen. This chapter positions '*Hamburger Queen* as a celebration of two embodied identities frequently undervalued in both heteronormative and queer culture, namely femme and fat'. Chalklin does this through a methodological approach she terms 'performance autoethnography' that combines being a performer in the competition and reflexive autoethnographic practices. She uses this chapter to reflect on her experience of being a finalist in the final *Hamburger Queen* and considers the radical potential of its 'camp trash aesthetics and ambiguous affect'. In this chapter, she argues that *Hamburger Queen* provided a deliberately provocative and controversial engagement with fat challenging the very normativities of the gender binary that reappear in both fat and LGBTQ subcultures. Chalklin urges readers to consider the radical potential of fat embodiment by, instead of resisting the 'obesity epidemic' rhetoric of the future of the fat body, choosing to 'exist in a parallel temporality that could be nothing but queer'.

The Pornography of Fat

As discussed earlier, this book includes original considerations of the ways in which pornography can potentially enable different forms of fat activism. This section examines fat pornography from the perspectives of both its performers and creators (see Ingraham's chapter) and its audience (see Chapter 9 by Smiet and Klumbyte). These chapters explore the complexities of representing fat bodies as sexual in a social and political climate that is openly hostile to their very existence.

Natalie Ingraham combines activism and academic research in her chapter 'Queering Porn: Gender and Size Diversity within SF Bay Area Queer Pornography'. She defines 'queer porn' as 'a genre that includes lesbian, gay, bisexual, trans*, queer or genderqueer (LGBTQ) performers, or creators (including directors or producers)'. Ingraham highlights that a key aspect of queer porn, according to the in-depth interviews with porn performers and creators, is their identity rather than the inclusion or exclusion of any specific sexual acts. This chapter focuses on the 'experiences of fat-identified performers and directors' from this queer porn community, paying particular attention to Courtney Trouble and Sophia St. James. Key areas of analysis include: the role of queer porn as a form of community, fat queer porn creating visibility and the activist politics that that entails, and its engagement with the feminist porn movement. Ingraham combines extensive quotations from the interviewees with analytical rigour to provide an insightful analysis of fat queer porn.

In 'Bodies like our own? The Dynamics of Distance and Closeness in Online Fat Porn,' Katrine Smiet and Goda Klumbyte offer a very different analytical approach to fat porn, combining feminist phenomenology with porn studies and new media approaches. They use phenomenology to consider the affective and often ambiguous responses of fat viewers to fat porn, and think about whether this affects a person's self image. They argue that 'body-image resonance [for the viewers] opens up spaces of potential as well as constraint in lived experience of fatness'. This ambivalent relationship to pornography raises broader questions for the authors about the impact of the online fat community and its effect in mediating sex for its members. Examples used to consider this claim come from the language and images that dominate fat porn, and from an analysis of an online column on fat sex by Tasha Fierce (as well as responses to this column). This section reflects upon a range of opinions on whether fat pornography online has activist potential.

Culturally (In)visible Bodies

The final section of the book brings fat studies, sexuality studies and literary studies together through three chapters that focus on specific representations of fat sex in literature. To help see the changes in the ways in which literature depicts fat sex we have organized these chapters in a chronological fashion, starting with research addressing writing from the early twentieth century, then the 1970s, and through to the early twenty-first century. Sarah Parker's chapter examines the relationship between food, the body and homoerotic desire in the poetry (and embodied personage) of Amy Lowell. Michelle Green's chapter moves the focus to Canada, where she examines Margaret Atwood's novel *Lady Oracle* (1976), and considers the ways in which its protagonist negotiates the fat woman's sexual double-bind (as simultaneously hypersexual and asexual). Laura Ellen Joyce's chapter offers a symbolic reading of fat sex in Blake Butler's *EVER* (2009), in which the house itself is a character, and explores questions of space, sexuality and desire.

In 'Amy Lowell's Appetites: Food, Consumption and Homoerotic Desire in Amy Lowell's Poetry', Sarah Parker offers a re-reading of Lowell's poetry with explicit reference to the pleasure that its author found in her physicality as a fat woman. Parker provides a close textual analysis of Lowell's love lyrics featured in *Pictures of the Floating World* (1919) – poems inspired by her long-term relationship with Ada Russell. Parker focuses on 'the connections between food, appetite and eroticism in Lowell's poetic work – looking at how Lowell frequently uses food imagery as a metaphor for sexual pleasure, and appetite as a metaphor for desire'. This symbolic analysis of fat sex provides a new lens to consider this poet's work – work that was often over-shadowed by her fat figure.

Rather than considering excess of desire and sexual appetite (as in Parker's reading of Lowell), Michelle Green instead focuses on their lack in her chapter 'Coming of Age through Weight Loss: The Fat Woman as Sexually Amature in Margaret Atwood's *Lady Oracle*'. Green examines 'the complex interchange between abjection, de-sexualisation and the subjectivity of the fat woman', specifically focusing on *Lady Oracle*'s fat female protagonist. To make this analytic move she coins the term 'sexual amaturity […] to refer to the negation of the character's social and sexual maturity', which provides new insight into a novel that has already been analysed by many Atwood scholars. She argues that *Lady Oracle* is the pioneer text of a subgenre of female coming-of-age novels that use weight loss to indicate psychological change. In addition to genre studies, Green draws on fat studies to offer new analysis of the character's sexuality and relationships with men throughout the novel. These combine to create an innovative interpretation of a key novel by Margaret Atwood that engages with the complex hypersexual/asexual fat female double bind that is a common trope in wider culture.

Laura Ellen Joyce's chapter 'Flesh Home: The Uncanny Female Architecture of Blake Butler's *EVER*' offers a symbolic interpretation of fat sex by focusing on the relationship between 'sexuality, flesh and spatiality'. Butler's novella sees the unnamed female protagonist fit into her home by becoming a part of the house, with both she and it constantly changing size. Joyce uses Freud's analysis of the uncanny and the discomfort surrounding female genitalia to analyse an experimental literary text which depicts 'an ontological wholeness – a fusion of flesh and home that is insoluble'. Joyce argues that in *EVER*, it is the juxtaposition of the suburban setting of the house and the way its architecture starts to take over the protagonist that creates the horror, which is reminiscent of Freud's analysis of the uncanny. Joyce explores themes of femininity and being engulfed, as well as the relationship between fat, mother and the womb, which together provides a symbolic interpretation of fat sex.

Creative Interludes

In this book, we wanted to follow in the footsteps of other largely academic collections that straddle similar activist-academic boundaries, such as *Fat Studies in the UK* (2009), *The Fat Studies Reader* (2009) and *Anarchism and Sexuality* (2011). This strategy enables us to include a wider variety of responses to the question of how to represent and discuss fat sex, from writers, academics, activists and para-academics. For the explicitly creative pieces, we have chosen to include a poem, a short story and a piece of autoethnographic writing, all interspersed between the more conventionally academic chapters. Alison Winch's poem 'Dumpling' explores the evocative and symbolic relationship between food, bodies and sensuality. Jennifer Lee and Kimberly Dark's pieces, meanwhile, move away from the symbolic and instead draw on embodied lived experiences of being fat to explore the interconnections between these experiences and sex and sexuality.

Jennifer Lee's powerful work of autoethnography in Chapter 7, 'Hidden and Forbidden: Alter Egos, Invisibility Cloaks and Psychic Fat Suits', explores how – through writing – she discovered that seemingly disparate parts of her life were connected. Lee's piece is a 'dance around the themes of fat, masculinities, sex and sexuality'. The reader follows Lee's journey in exploring her sexuality from shame filled teenage experiences to casual sexual encounters, culminating with the discovery of ways to enjoy inhabiting her fat body. It is a vital contribution to the collection because it is the only chapter of the book that explicitly engages with masculinities and the journey of self-discovery that seems fundamental to many narratives that dominate the fatosphere.

In the final chapter, Kimberly Dark's short story-come-essay, entitled 'Coming Out Fat', provides a complex critique of the ways in which fat and sexuality impact on both parties in a relationship. Dark uses the creative format to explore the fat lived experience of inhabiting a socially marginalized and discriminated against identity and body. She encourages her lovers to consider how they feel about being with a fat beautiful woman who feels happy in her skin when society and their friends argue that she should change. While Dark's piece might be short, we chose it to close the book because it helps explore some big questions.

The materials that are gathered here are wide-ranging in their content and disciplinary perspectives, allowing for a lot of diverse ground to be covered. However, there are still dimensions to the issue of fat sex that do not receive the close attention they deserve. Detailed debates about masculinities, for example, are notable by their absence (though they are discussed in Chapter 7), and the editors would have liked to have included more material dedicated to discussing the ways in which race impacts on the perception, representation and embodied experiences of fat women of colour. As we identified at the beginning of this introduction, intersectional approaches to fat embodiment have been a hallmark of much of the excellent work produced under the umbrella term of fat studies, and it is disappointing to be unable to offer a more complete reflection of this here. However, as more critical attention is given to the issues of sex and sexuality within fat studies we are confident that material will be produced that addresses these blind spots and helps to round out our understanding. In bringing together voices from across the spectrum of academia and activism, *Fat Sex: New Directions in Theory and Activism* will, we hope, make an original contribution both to sexuality studies and to the emerging area of fat studies, extending existing research and staging a timely intervention into the field while offering a new point of departure for contemporary debate.

The chapters in *Fat Sex*, while tackling the question from a range of disciplinary, stylistic and theoretical approaches, all want to dismantle the idea that fat and sex should not and do not mesh. They want to change the way that (fat) people and scholars themselves think and feel about fat sex. In this volume, fat sex is shown to flourish and engage with the very social and cultural forces claiming it to be abhorrent. The collection demonstrates ways that activism, academic study and lived experience inform one another. By assembling the chapters in this book we hope to highlight some of the productive tensions that emerge when fat studies and sexuality studies meet. With *Fat Sex* we hope to disrupt received notions about the interplay between fat, gender and sex and to encourage further examination of fat sex.

References

Blank, H. 2011. *Big Big Love, Revised: A Sex and Relationships Guide for People of Size*, revised edn, Celestial Arts, Berkeley.

Cooper, C. 2009. 'Maybe it should be called Fat American Studies', *The Fat Studies Reader*, eds. Rothblum, E., and Solovay, S., New York University Press, New York and London, pp. 327–333.

Dury, S. and Thorp, S. 1994. *Viz, The Big Fat Slags Book*, John Brown Publishing.

'Fat and How Not to Be: The Cause (or the problem with hippies ...)', n.d. *Everybody Sucks But Me*, zine.
FaT GiRL Collective. (1994–1997). *FaT GiRL: A Zine for Fat Dykes and the Women Who Want Them, #1–7,* Fat Girl Publishing, San Francisco.
'Fat is so COOL', n.d. *I'm So Fucking Beautiful*, zine, no. 1
'Fat Oppression and Fat Liberation', 1991. *Three Dollar Bill*, zine, no. 1.
'fatfatfatfatfat', n.d. *The Nerdy Grrrl Revolution*, zine, no. 1.
fat-sex.tumblr.com [WWW Document], n.d. URL http://fat-sex.tumblr.com/ (accessed 25/5/14).
fatsexadvice.tumblr.com [WWW Document], n.d. URL http://fatsexadvice.tumblr.com/?og=1 (accessed 25/5/14).
fat-sex-is-good-sex.tumblr.com [WWW Document], n.d. URL http://fat-sex-is-good-sex.tumblr.com/ (accessed 25/5/14).
Gailey, J. and Proshaska, A., 2006. '"Knocking off a Fat Girl": an Exploration of Hogging, Male Sexuality, and Neutralizations', *Deviant Behaviour*, 27:1, 31–49.
Heckert, J. and Cleminsen, R. 2011. *Sexuality and Anarchism: Ethics, Relationships and Power.* Routledge, London and New York.
Lupton, D. 2012. *Fat*, Routledge, Abingdon and New York.
Murray, S. 2004. 'Locating Aesthetics: Sexing the Fat Woman', *Social Semiotics*, 14:3, 237–247.
Pausé, C., Wykes, J., and Murray, S. (eds). 2014. *Queering Fat Embodiment*, Ashgate, Farnham.
Rothblum, E., and Solovay, S. (eds) 2009. *The Fat Studies Reader*, New York University Press, New York and London.
Scottee (2014a). Happy Fatties are Erased from the Media [Online] Available: http://www.feministtimes.com/happy-fatties-are-erased-from-the-media/ (accessed 19/06/14).
Snider, S. 2009. 'Alternative Publications and the Visualizing of Fat and Queer Eroto-politics in Contemporary American Culture', *The Fat Studies Reader*, eds. Rothblum, E., and Solovay, S., New York University Press, New York and London, pp. 223–230.
The Adventures of Big Girl, 1993, zine, no. 1.
Tomrley, C. and Naylor, A.K. (eds) 2009. *Fat Studies in the UK*, Raw Nerve Books, York.
Tovar, V., 2012. *Hot and Heavy: Fierce Fat Girls on Life, Love & Fashion*, Seal Press, Berkeley.
Weinstein, R.J, 2012. *Fat Sex: The Naked Truth*, CreateSpace Independent Publishing Platform, North Charleston.

Fat Histories, Fat Communities

Chapter 2
Fat as a Feminist Issue: A History

Zora Simic

In 2013 the thirtieth anniversary of the 1983 publication of the anthology *Shadow on a Tightrope*, a collection of writings by women on fat oppression, was cause for much celebration in the 'fatosphere'. Ragen Chastain, founder of the online archive *In Our Own Words: A Fat Activist History*, was a young girl when *Shadows* was first published, and marvelled at 'how these women came together – without the internet, the fatsophere, facebook or smartphones' to help start a 'movement from scratch' (Chastain, 2013). Fat Studies pioneer Esther Rothblum cited *Shadows* as a 'classic book' that by that early 1990s was one of 'over a dozen' fat affirmative books available. In the past decade Rothblum has established the *Fat Studies* journal, co-edited the *Fat Studies Reader* (2011) and her first edition of *Shadows* is worn from re-reading (Rothblum, 2013). British fat activist, psychotherapist and writer Charlotte Cooper, ever attentive to the US-centrism of fat politics, also owns a 'dog-eared' copy that she treasures, but hers is from 1989 when *Shadow* was first published in Britain. She bought her copy in the feminist bookshop Silver Moon, and is both 'grateful for' and 'wary of' the 'feminist sensibility' that produced and disseminated *Shadow* in the first place: that is 'essentialist, fundamentalist and separatist feminisms' that have since been meaningfully critiqued and challenged by people of colour, trans people, queers, sex positive feminists and sex workers. Still, it was not necessary to be part of US lesbian feminism to appreciate it: 'I had the vital knowledge of my own fat body, and *Shadow on a Tightrope* validated that knowledge' (Cooper, 2013).

This short survey of responses to *Shadow*'s thirtieth birthday is a mere sample of a much larger corpus of commemoration which collectively illustrates a growing historical consciousness within fat activist communities, eager to affirm their politics through the creation of a historical tradition. While not all fat activists are women (though more are than not) and not all women within fat activism are feminists (though feminism's influence on fat politics is obvious) this chapter is more focused on fat activists who *do* identify as feminist, both past and present, though there is hardly room to do proper justice to a history of fat feminist activism that now spans decades, continents, alliances and a variety of feminisms. I am also concerned with how feminism generally has addressed fat within its politics. In particular, I will consider how fat sex and sexuality have been incorporated (or not) into a feminist politics of fat, from a variety of standpoints, including the personal (as in some of the essays in *Shadow*) and the interpretative (such as Susie Orbach's psycho-social reading of fat or disordered eating as a possible rejection of society's shifting expectations of female sexuality).

I seek to bring these two histories together for several reasons. Firstly, fat activism forms part of the longer history of feminist body politics that dates back at least as far as the mid-nineteenth century when British and North American women activists pursued dress reform. Yet histories of feminism tend to overlook or marginalise fat activism and its contribution to feminist body politics. For example, in her ambitious history of modern feminism, *No Turning Back* (2002) Estelle B. Freedman gives coverage to the now iconic protest against the Miss America pageant in 1968 and the rise of the women's health movement, but does not mention Fat Underground, the originators of fat liberation.

Secondly, and relatedly, fat activism was a vibrant part of second-wave feminism (more specifically women's liberation, radical feminism and lesbian feminism) and third-wave feminism and constitutes one of the most dynamic and creative arenas of feminist and queer activism in the present.

And thirdly, and most importantly, fat has been identified as part of the unfinished business of feminism (Chrisler, 2012). The alleged signs of feminism's failure on this front are most obviously indicated by the enduring female commitment to regimes of beautification (for example, dieting) and an abiding fatphobia that is arguably most prevalent in those societies in which feminism has achieved the most success and influence. Indeed some have suggested that contemporary understandings of fat (especially female fat) as undesirable, unhealthy and transgressive share an historical emergence with modern feminism, with fatphobia or fat stigma and its corollary the cult of thinness, part of a wider backlash against the advance of women's rights (Wolf, 1991, p. 184). In any case, there is historical consensus that the desire to be thin and the rise of dieting culture manifest at the turn of the nineteenth to the twentieth century in western societies, beginning with the white middle classes and across the gender divide, though it was women who faced disproportionate pressure to subscribe to the new slim ideal, with anti-fat attitudes assuming a distinctly misogynist character from the 1920s (Stearns, 1997).

While acknowledging that it is hardly possible for feminism to challenge and eradicate these pervasive features of modern life on its own, some critics have identified and implicated an enduring feminist ambivalence about fat and its meanings as a barrier to a proper feminist intervention into not only heteronormative beauty culture, its institutions and its effects, but also the alleged obesity 'epidemic' (Kirkland, 2011). To ponder these charges against feminism, this chapter brings together two histories that reveal both the extent and limits of a feminist fat politics so far.

First I focus on the development of fat feminism, from the Fat Underground through to the queer fat activism of the FaT GiRL collective in the 1990s and in the 'fatosphere' in the present. Next I trace mainstream feminist critiques of fat via best-selling texts such as Susie Orbach's *Fat is a Feminist* Issue (1978) and *The Beauty Myth* by Naomi Wolf (1991) and a selection of writings from the 'third wave' of US feminism. While there are obvious limits to presenting Orbach and Wolf and their texts as representative of feminism, particularly at a grass roots level, their influence (for better or worse) cannot be denied, particularly Orbach whose book title has been widely paraphrased as the point of origin for a feminist discussion of fat, including by people who admit to not having read the book. Lastly, I briefly consider the status of fat as a contemporary feminist issue and the place of sex within this, while also reiterating the spaces that various feminisms opened up to address and envision 'fat sex'. Across these sections, 'sexual politics' is broadly interpreted in order to capture the variety of ways sex has manifested in fat activism and in its intersections with feminist and queer movements. Since the late 1960s, fat activists and feminists have consistently and creatively politicised the personal, including embodiment and sexual pleasure, and it is not surprising that a specifically *feminist* fat activism emerged in the early years of Women's Liberation. Yet, as will be demonstrated, the issues of fat sex and sexuality have had the capacity – in the past and into the present – to call into question the obvious affinities between fat activism and feminism.

Throughout, the terms 'fat feminism' and '[second/third wave] feminism' are deployed heuristically rather than definitively. The purpose is not to quarantine one form from the other: I present these inevitably sweeping histories as partial, distinct and intersecting, with an emphasis on moments of convergence between fat activism and feminism; interactions between and within them have been both productive and fraught, and are indicative of the different forms and orientations of both fat activism and feminism. In pursuit of progressive sexual politics, some fat activists have emphasised their affinity with queer over feminism, while others have identified fatphobic attitudes within feminism and queer respectively. More common is aligning the three: Fat, feminism and queer. It is at this intersection that the theme of sex is often most fruitfully explored, as will emerge in this chapter.

Fat Feminism

Fat activism is typically dated to the late 1960s in the United States, when a series of isolated protests against the dominant medical and social models of fat culminated in the formation of the National Association to Aid Fat Americans in 1969, now the National Association to Advance Fat Acceptance

(NAAFA). NAAFA's activities, however, were mostly social rather than political and its participants continue to include male 'fat admirers' seeking fat women as sexual partners. Research has revealed a spectrum of negative to positive experiences between fat women and 'FAs' (Goode and Priessler, 1983), but it is hardly surprising that their presence in fat communities partly contributed to the emergence of an explicitly feminist fat activism that distinguished itself from NAAFA through its more confrontational mode of activism and its location within lesbian feminism. The Fat Underground, a collective drawn from radical therapy and radical feminist circles, emerged in southern California in the early 1970s after two of its founders, Sara Fishman (also known as Aldebaran and Vivian F. Mayer) and Judy Freespirit split from NAAFA. Together they wrote the 'Fat Manifesto' in late 1973, which circulated in various feminist publications throughout the second half of the 1970s, before being re-published in *Shadow* in 1983.

From its inception, the feminist fat liberation movement distinguished itself from other forms of fat activism on the basis of its 'cogent and radical analysis of fat oppression' (Mayer, 1983, p. x) and its links with 'the struggles of other oppressed groups against classism, racism, sexism, ageism, capitalism, imperialism and the like', to quote the Fat Manifesto (Freespirit and Alderbaran, 1983, p. 53). The cross-pollination of ideas and political struggles of the late 1960s and early 1970s were evident in the Manifesto's concluding words, an inspired revision of a classic Marxist slogan: 'FAT PEOPLE OF THE WORLD, UNITE! YOU HAVE *NOTHING* TO LOSE … '.

Within the lesbian feminist milieu of LA, the Fat Underground, originally only a handful of people, formed the core of feminist fat liberation. At the Women's Equality Day celebration in August 1974 the movement made their public debut: a vigil for recently deceased singer 'Mama' Cass Elliot (Mayer, 1983, p. xiv). Despite rumours she had choked to death on a ham sandwich, Mama Cass had died of a heart attack most likely caused by a fasting diet (Farrell, 2011, p. 144). The Fat Underground's Lynn Mabel-Lois, a medical librarian who penned much of the movement's anti-diet literature, took to the stage to celebrate Cass as a 'fat woman who refused to hide her beauty' and to accuse the medical establishment of 'committing genocide against women'. In the afterglow, among their peers, the activists were 'local heroines' (Fishman, 1998). Fat Underground held workshops, produced more literature, staged protests outside weight loss clinics and aligned with other feminist causes, including one memorable occasion in 1975 where as part of a rally protesting crimes against women, Mabel-Lois denounced weight-loss surgery and starvation diets as part of a world-wide pattern of violence 'based on sexism' (Mayer, 1983, p. xv).

By the mid-1970s, fat feminism was also developing on the east coast of the US: activist Karen Scott-Jones (later Karen Stimson), part of a 'Feminist Caucus' in NAAFA, got in touch with the Fat Underground and in 1975 wrote the first essays on fat feminism for her local National Council of Women (NOW) newsletter and for NAAFA, the latter 'a primer on the relationship of sexism to size-ism' (Stimson, n.d 2). When original Fat Underground members Alderbaran (also and later known as Vivian Mayer) and Sharon Bas Hannah moved east, they formed the Fat Liberation Front with Stimson, making New Haven Connecticut an emerging centre of fat activism. From there, Mayer started Fat Liberator Publications in 1978 as a means of disseminating literature and in doing so broke down some of the isolation that had hitherto obstructed a national fat liberation movement. Both Mayer and Stimson recalled 1980 as a turning point, with the first national conference of fat feminist activists – 17 in all – held in April (Mayer, 1983, p. xvi); shortly after, Judith Stein of Boston Fat Liberation successfully lobbied the publishing collective of the iconic tome of the feminist health movement *Our Bodies, Ourselves* to revise its anti-fat and pro-diet stance, and to include fat liberation resources (Stimson, n.d 3). In this consolidating phase of fat liberation, its energies were as directed to raising awareness of fat politics within feminism as to fighting fat oppression and discrimination in wider society and its institutions.

Later, Mayer described how important the blossoming lesbian feminist community in LA had been to the fat liberationists:

> The companionship of other women offered fat women a social environment in which – often for the first time in their lives – they could be loved for their intelligence and their personalities, and their 'ugliness' according to conventional standards could be overlooked. Indeed, these conventional standards were attacked as oppressive to women. In theory ... lesbian feminism offered a haven wherein a fat woman could affirm her beleaguered sense of womanhood and could almost forget she was fat. (Mayer, 1983, p. xiv)

Yet if radical feminism offered a language through which to understand fat oppression as a feature of patriarchal capitalist societies in which fat hatred was disproportionately directed at women, evidence of fatphobia *within* lesbian feminism (whether it be slim lesbians rejecting fat women as lovers, offering unsolicited weight loss advice or failing to adequately incorporate fat oppression into their feminism) 'helped sort out issues of fat politics versus generalized sexism' (Mayer, 1983, p. xiv). By the time *Shadow* was published in 1983 – by new feminist press Aunt Lute Books and edited by Lisa Schoenfielder and Barb Weiser – negative or disappointing experiences of anti-fat attitudes in the women's movement featured in numerous accounts.

The writer Elana Dykewomon, celebrated in lesbian feminist circles following the publication of her 1974 novel *Riverfinger Woman*, wrote in her essay 'Travelling Fat' of the daily grind of 'fat womyn trying to be part of community', of fat liberation workshops at feminist conferences where the first hour was taken up 'struggling with the old myths about fat womyn, especially that fat womyn aren't healthy, and couldn't expect to have enjoyable sexual experiences' (Dykewomon 1983, p. 146). Dykewomon began to speak up, interjecting fat politics into discussions of Chinese footbinding by drawing parallels with diet regimes and class mobility. All the while, she pursued her fantasy of 'fat dykes everywhere', involved and affirmed in the wider movement. But the fat dykes she did meet were usually as isolated and frustrated as herself, their fat politics dismissed as bourgeois and indulgent (Dykewomon, 1983, p. 150). As its republication in *Shadow* suggested, it appeared little had changed since 1975 when Laurie Ann Lepoff first published her essay 'Fat Politics' and declared she felt 'more solidarity with a fat suburban housewife than I do with my slender lesbian sisters' (Lepoff, 1983, p. 205).

Still, if lesbian feminism could not be as accommodating to fat activists as they wished it to be, fat liberation's own location within it left it open to its charges of exclusivity. Indeed, the editors of *Shadow* expressed concern that their anthology 'doesn't speak often enough to fat women who survive without the support of political communities' (Schoenfielder and Wieser, 1983, p. xxi). And while the 35 chapters are mostly from the position of white, middle-class lesbians involved in fat liberation and lesbian feminism, the anthology did not lack in diversity: points of view were gathered from fat women of colour, in high school, in heterosexual relationships, who were aging or working-class or in a wheelchair or in the case of 'Nancy' from the perspective of a woman suffering from both bulimia and anorexia. Nancy's interview allowed the editors to make explicit connections between fat oppression and fat hatred and eating disorders and to condemn feminism for not taking this connection seriously (Schoenfielder and Wieser, 1983, p. 179). Throughout contributors provided material evidence of fat oppression and situated the fat woman and her treatment as paradigmatic of women everywhere. Women's fear of fat, argued Fat Underground, 'is a means of social control against women', and the position of fat women reveals 'the true position of women in our society': as sexual objects whose sexuality is taken away from them or presumably forfeited when a woman is fat (Mabel-Lois and Aldebaran, 1983, pp. 54–5).

Karen Scott-Jones' presence in Fat Liberation, and her contribution to *Shadow*, the essay 'Attraction and/or Intimidation: Fat Women's Sexual Dilemmas' also complicate any assessment of Fat Liberation as exclusively lesbian feminist. A virgin until she was 26, Scott-Jones was galvanised into fat activism after reading about a man who loved fat women: 'Reading about his sexual experiences with them felt like the force of a bombshell exploding inside me. The women he wrote about making love with were my size and bigger!' (Scott-Jones, 1983, p. 216). Part of her politicisation as a fat feminist was realising how her anger and frustration 'was directly related to fat women's status as sexual pariahs' (p. 217). Another part was experimenting sexually with various Fat Admirers she met through NAAFA. 'But the rampant sexism among the men I encountered offended me', she wrote, 'as did the options they seemed to be offering', i.e. one-night stands or affairs. She resented those men seeking to accumulate 'conquests' and their assumption that fat women would be grateful for the attention. Further:

> [N]one of these men's apparent notions about fat women's sexual identity seemed to fit mine: I was neither so perpetually horny I'd go to bed with any man, anytime, nor an Earth mother type, nor a totally 'feminine' woman bent solely on pleasing a man: I was simply a young fat woman looking for a male person with whom I could develop a relationship. (Scott-Jones, p. 218)

At the time of writing, Scott-Jones was 'relationshipless-by-choice' and talking and thinking about fat sex and sexuality in her fat woman's support group in which their meetings 'often returned to sex-related issues no matter what topic we may be discussing' (p. 221). Later, she would marry Richard Stimson, a Fat Admirer, and the couple co-founded Largesse: The Network for Size Esteem. She also remained very active in fat feminism and routinely targeted mainstream feminism for neglecting fat women and/or abetting fatphobia by valourising thin-ness (Stimson, 2008).

Loraine Hutchins, in a generally positive review of *Shadow* published in radical feminist journal *off our backs* in 1985, was most responsive to those essays that relayed everyday fat embodiment: the lovers who come and go, the joy and struggle of exercise, the grind of finding clothes to fit and flatter, the navigation of public spaces and judgment and the pain and consequences of diets, pharmaceuticals and surgeries prescribed by doctors. Scott-Jones' essay was singled out as especially resonant with her account of her sex life read as symptomatic of general 'sexual dilemmas' for fat women, who are simultaneously conflated with sex and eroticism and rejected as desirable sexual partners (Hutchins, 1985, p. 24). Hutchins was less enthused about the 'defence of fat' running through the collection, manifested in an anti-diet stance that taken as a whole, she argued, was 'just not true'. Missing too was proper examination of compulsive eating, or any proposed feminist solutions to it (p. 25). This is a fault-line that remains in fat feminism: how to live or embody your fat feminist politics (Murray, 2005).

In the decade Hutchins reviewed *Shadow* she was also developing her own feminist sexual politics, namely bisexual feminism, which she championed in her 'Biatribe' published in *off our backs* in 1988. Here, Hutchins affirmed a sex positive feminism she positioned as the antithesis of the 'erotophobia' of the feminist sex wars and the backlash against the HIV-AIDS crisis (Hutchins, 1988). With another fat-identified feminist Lani Ka'ahumanu, Hutchins edited the anthology *Bi Any Other Name: Bisexual People Speak Out* (1991), which is as foundational to bisexual politics as *Shadow* is to fat feminism. In 1994, Ka'ahumanu was among the 41 women photographed nude and in situ by Laurie Toby Edison for *Women En Large: Images of Fat Nudes* (Edison and Notkin, 1994). This book has since been credited with bringing fat acceptance and positivity to mainstream attention (Snider, 2012) and is also representative of the broader sex-focused and sex positive activism of Hutchins and Ka'ahumanu who rarely feature in historical accounts of fat feminism. This is not surprising given that they were not especially active in Fat Liberation, yet their activism offers another route by which fat has been meaningfully incorporated into feminist sexual politics.

Meanwhile, Fat liberation continued into the 1980s, as part of radical (or 'cultural') feminism in the United States. In stops and starts, fat feminism was also manifesting outside of the US, most notably in Holland, France and in the UK, where in a landmark edition of *Spare Rib* in 1987 fat liberation was put on the cover of the magazine and on the agenda of British women's liberation. Tina Jenkins and Heather Smith – partly drawing on *Shadow* and various Fat Liberator publications – insisted fat oppression be properly recognised as a feminist issue, implored fat feminists to organise collectively to put fat oppression on the wider political agenda as activists had in the US, and pre-empting the rise of fat positivity, argued that '[f]at women must eventually move beyond the analysis of how bad things are to a celebration of ourselves' (Jenkins and Smith, 1987 pp. 14–18). Here, British fat liberationists were signalling a shift to fat positivity, which as it would develop in the 1990s was increasingly focused on celebrating the fat female body as desirable and desiring and/or queer insofar as sexy fat bodies defy normative understandings of female sex appeal and behaviour.

The 'queer turn' in fat feminist politics was also prefigured by the emergence of the pioneering Fat Lip Readers Theatre group, founded in the 1980s by a group of fat activists that included Judy Freespirit, some of whom also had disabilities, making explicit connections between fat and disabled embodiment and experience in their performances. In June 1990, the defiantly fat-positive Fat Dykes of San Francisco marched down Castro Street to launch their first 'Let It All Hang Out Day' as a protest against anti-fat and anti-dyke material in the local press. Fat queer and trans people have been an important part of fat activism since its inception (Cooper, 2011, p. 7), while fat activism also shared members with vanguard queer collectives such as Queer Nation and Lesbian Avengers.

Without wanting to insist on too neat a rupture between gay and queer politics, the ascent of queer theory and activism in the 1990s reinvigorated and in some cases redirected fat feminist politics. Like gay liberation, fat liberation had throughout the 1970s and into the 1980s drawn on influential theories of stigma, oppression and deviance to develop its political vocabulary and critique, and both movements encouraged 'coming out' to reclaim and positively occupy a stigmatised identity. If the 'coming out' narrative still seems less applicable to fat bodies or has its limits (Murray, 2005, p. 270), its endurance within fat feminism offers evidence of its salience as a de-stigmatising strategy, as a source of fat positivity and of a shared history with gay and lesbian movements (Saguy and Ward, 2011, p. 11).

What queer offered – and indeed shared with – fat liberation groups were practices of subversion and spectacle, in which gender, sexuality and fat were deconstructed in order to reveal and unsettle their socially and culturally constructed meanings, often via the body itself. For Heather McAllister, founder and director of Big Burlesque and the Fat-Bottom Revue in the late 1990s, the fat liberation she first encountered reading *Shadow* could only properly manifest when she experienced it 'physically as well as accepting it politically and theoretically' (McAllister, 2009, p. 305). For McAllister, what distinguished her troupes as queer in the wider neo-burlesque scene, was their commitment to fat liberation. All the dancers were fat, but beyond this exhibited a diverse range of gender identities, shapes, and abilities, 'with varying levels of comfort around strip tease and nudity' (p. 306). Some fat feminists were critical of what they perceived to be 'too much of a focus on sexuality', continued McAllister, but they were missing the point: fat liberation offered no freedom if it was only meant to apply from the 'neck up' (p. 311).

McAllister's sex positivity and focus on embodiment marked her fat activism as both queer and third-wave feminist, though as with radical lesbian feminism in the 1970s and 1980s, queer was not uniformly accommodating of fat activism or fat bodies, nor was queer theory's critique of identity politics necessarily compatible with fat activism. To better understand what 'queer' is at work in fat activism, LeBesco has described queer fat activism as performative, focussed more on 'repositioning fat in the cultural imaginary' than on policy (LeBesco, 2001, p. 83), while Cooper uses queer in relation to fat activism 'as an umbrella term for lesbians and dykes and questioning and transgressive women rather than Bears, who have a different political trajectory'. She also means 'feminists, by and large' (Cooper, 2011, p. 7).

In Stefanie Snider's analyses of the mid-1990s zine series *FaT GiRL: A Zine for Fat Dykes and the Women who want them*, produced by the San Francisco-based FaT GiRL Collective, she notes that the Collective's use of sexually explicit photographs to foreground the sexual desirability of fat dykes drew on 'visual cues from traditional and feminist pornographic imagery' in service of a fat queer politics that owed much to 'the 1970s feminist stance that the personal is political' (Snider, 2010, p. 182). Sexy pictures of fat women enjoying sex and food, often both at once, also challenged dominant representations of the fat body as abject, as false (not yet thin) or past (once was fat), rather than embodied and present (Kent, 2001, p. 137). As with McAllister's embodied fat activism, the FaT GiRL Collective and their allies made sex and sexuality central to their politics without disavowing earlier Fat Liberation: the first issue included an interview with Judy Freespirit and various contributors cited *Shadow* as a foundational text (Kent, 2001, p. 138). The sometimes exaggerated but nevertheless discernible generational divide that marked out second from third wave feminism has not been as marked in fat feminism.

Where the waves model of feminist history has been applicable to fat feminism is in comprehending its peaks and troughs (Cooper, 2008). Fat Liberation never entirely disappeared, but fat feminism has clearly been more visible since the 1990s. The political strategies of queer, left-leaning punk (or queer core) and third-wave feminism (and their various sub-cultural manifestations) added new foci (including sex and sexuality) and constituents, who were now more likely to be exchanging ideas via the internet than at annual conferences.

By the turn of the millennium, fat feminism had its own celebrities, including Nomy Lamm and Marilyn Wann, respective founders of the zines *I'm So Fucking Beautiful* and *Fat? So!*, both of whom demand their right to sexual pleasure and reject prevailing stereotypes about fat women and desire. Wann's upbeat fat positivity, humour and creativity have earned her many fans, though her high profile has also meant her work has been used as an example of some of the limits of fat affirmation as a strategy for combating systemic and internalised fatphobia (Murray, 2005), including in or as a barrier to sexual and romantic relationships. In extolling the joys of fat sex, for example, Wann arguably reduces the complexity of fat sexualities to a series of feel-good assurances: fat women are more orgasmic than thin ones, that 'hard bodies are nice, but soft bodies are nicer' and that by loving your thighs 'you make it tough for anyone to hate them' (Wann, 1998, p. 178). Yet it is also the case that Wann speaks to multiple audiences, including young fat women who are disenfranchised politically or not especially interested in fat politics but are nevertheless drawn to Wann's empathetic writings, the Health At Every Size Movement of which she is a tireless champion and various experts within the interdisciplinary field of Fat Studies.

For Nony Lamm, meanwhile, reading *Shadow* had galvanised her to start her own zine *I'm So Fucking Beautiful* in 1991: in its xero-ed pages, Lamm directly addressed the hypothetical reader in possession of 'thin privilege', catalogued fatphobia in the punk scene she was part of, challenged any assumption that as a fat woman she was lacking in fashion sense and laid claim to a distinctly sexual fat queer identity. Her confessional style and intersectional politics made Lamm a popular figure in third-wave feminism, but it is important to note that her fat politics was also born of a rejection of 'mainstream feminist authors, who claim to be dealing with this issue, [but] are doing it in a very wrong way', i.e. by acknowledging fat oppression while also preaching the weight-loss benefits of healthy lifestyle and entertaining 'liberal' theories of fat as having its origins in psychological disturbance (Lamm, 1995). As Lamm told *Ms* magazine in 1997, the 'consumate example' of this 'bullshit' mainstream feminist view is

Susie Orbach's *Fat is a Feminist Issue*. With this rejection, Lamm continued an ongoing fat feminist critique of Orbach's theorising as reproducing rather than challenging dominant stereotypes about fat women – including the idea that fat women are "'compulsive overeaters", desperate for "protection, sex, mothering, strength, assertion and love"' (Higginbotham, 1997, p. 63).

Feminism and Fat

Susie Orbach was hardly the first second-wave feminist to bring women's bodies into focus, but her innovation was to bring feminism directly into the lives of women unhappy with and/or disconnected from their bodies. *Fat is a Feminist Issue* (*FIFI*), first published in 1978 and revised and reissued a number of times since (most recently in 2006), was a genuine trail-blazer, bringing to feminist and popular consciousness, female experiences of body hatred, disordered or compulsive eating and the western prejudice against fat and female fat in particular. It received widespread media attention, spawned a sequel and many women, especially those with personal histories of eating disorders, were empowered by Orbach's approach.

FIFI, pitched as a 'self-help manual', made bold claims that '[f]eminism argues that being fat represents an attempt to break free of society's sex stereotypes' and that fat is 'a response to the inequality of the sexes' (Orbach, 2006, p. 15). Women are encouraged to 'own' their fat – by working out its origins and functions – before they can break their addictive relationship to food and lose weight (86). If weight-loss is not the point of *FIFI*, it is certainly a by-product of a successful therapeutic and feminist analysis of one's fat. This message was augmented by before and after sketches of an archetypal woman who begins therapy with a layer of fat that acts as a barrier between herself and the world: as she addresses her fat, negative self-image and compulsive eating, the fat melts away to reveal the authentic slimmer self (Orbach, 2006, p. 84).

Not surprisingly, some of the most damning critiques of *FIFI* emerged from Fat Liberation. For Joan Dickenson, Orbach undermined her 'sound theory about women and fat' (Dickenson, 1983, p. 39) by reproducing blame-the-victim clichés such as fat women fear sex or 'crave size because women are powerless in this society' (p. 40). Further, in her lack of attention to economics and issues of race and class and focus on self-help, Orbach did little to dislodge the idea that fat is a personal problem rather than a societal one. British Fat Liberationists Tina Jenkins and Heather Smith questioned Orbach's assumption that 'all fat people eat compulsively, that all fat people who eat compulsively will become thin when they stop doing so, and that our fat makes us automatically either physically or mentally ill' (Jenkins and Smith, 1987, p. 16). In response, Orbach applauded the arrival of Fat Liberation to the UK while rejecting any claims that her work is 'an attack on fat' or assumes all fat women are compulsive eaters (Orbach, 1987, p. 4).

Orbach was still defending her approach in feminist journals into the 1980s, notably against Nicky Diamond's charge in *Feminist Review* that *FIFI* adheres to a fat/ thin binary in which the latter is endorsed in positive terms and that opportunities were missed to recognise the 'thin true sexual body' (for example) as a product of power relations and social construction (Diamond, 1985, p. 55). Orbach rejected the view that *FIFI* was 'anti-feminist' and staked a claim for her therapeutic approach as rooted in '*felt* experiences' in opposition to Diamond's preference for 'philosophical paradigms', an implicit reference to Diamond's use of Foucault to frame her critique (Orbach, 1985, pp. 120–21).

For Diamond, writing in 1985, it was the aspirational and normative power of 'thin' that was most urgently in need of feminist attention rather than 'fat'. Kim Chernin had already started this work, motivated by both her feminism and her own experience of eating disorders, first in *The Obsession: Reflections on the Tyranny of Slenderness* (1981), followed by *The Hungry Self: Women, Eating and Identity* (1985) and *Reinventing Eve: Modern Woman in Search of Herself* (1987). By the 1990s, female commitment to the slender body ideal – especially as manifested in bulimia and anorexia nervosa – was the locus of concern for an increasing number of feminists, most notably Naomi Wolf in her blockbuster debut *The Beauty Myth* (1990), one of the inaugurating texts of third wave feminism, and feminist philosopher Susan Bordo who launched an identifiable field of feminist body studies with her Pulitzer-prize nominated 1993 book *Unbearable Weight: Feminism, Western Culture, and the Body*. These swiftly influential texts were each distinctively ambitious and oriented, but both shared the view that the unprecedented rates of bulimia and anorexia nervosa amongst girls and women in western societies in the 1980s required more than a medical explanation: as mass phenomena they demanded cultural and feminist analysis. Anorexia, wrote Wolf, is to the late twentieth-century what hysteria was to the Victorian era (Wolf, 1991, p. 198), an 'ideology of semistarvation [that] undoes feminism' (p. 96) and repudiates female sexuality by asking women to shed the fat that makes them fertile, desirable and desiring (p. 193). The hungry dieting woman is 'politically castrate', too depleted of energy 'to get angry or get organised, or to chase sex' (p. 199). For Bordo, eating disorders analysed as a 'social phenomenon rather than personal pathology, represented a crystallisation' of historical and contemporary currents in Western culture (Bordo, 2003, p. xxi). And the 'starving white girls', she wrote in her introduction to the tenth anniversary edition, 'were just the forward guard, the miners' canaries warning how poisonous the air was becoming for everyone' (p. xx).

The writings of Wolf, Bordo and others were in response to an identifiable upsurge or epidemic of eating disorders and their influence travelled in a number of directions as feminism was further institutionalised in the academy while also revived in popular consciousness. Wolf's *The Beauty Myth* was so successful that she gave third wave feminism an identifiable spokesperson and one of its most obvious causes in a packed and eclectic agenda: eating disorders and body image. A spate of studies, memoirs and anthologies focused on young women's bodies and their vulnerabilities followed (Baumgardner and Richards, 2000, p. 21), including the 1998 anthology *Adiós, Barbie: Young women write about Body Image and Identity* (republished in 2000 as *Body Outlaws*) that featured among its diverse range of contributors Nomy Lamm and plus-sized model Kate Dillon. Consistent with the third wave's pro-sex intersectional politics and its preference for first-person narratives, several contributors explicitly linked their body and sexual politics ('I'm a fat, sleazy, one-legged, anarchist dyke, and I'm a total hottie', declared Lamm 2003, p. 82), while the editors insisted on a broader definition of 'body image' that encompassed skin colour, hair texture, eye colour, facial features and other physical markers of ethnic and racial difference. The identification of body weight as a white girl's issue was also confounded by the personal experiences of women such as Regina D. Williams, size acceptance activist and the first African American chairperson of the Michigan chapter of NAAFA. As African Americans became more assimilated 'into mainstream society' and its 'Eurocentric standards of beauty', wrote Williams, 'our "Big Mamas"' [who] 'were once considered women of beauty and strength' are now 'a source of embarrassment, the object of cruel remarks and constant harassment about their weight' (Williams, 2003, p. 183). Taken together, the essays in *Body Outlaws* and other third wave anthologies exemplified a 'critical form of embodied politics' that advocated 'personal, bodily resistance to oppressive ideologies' (Fixmer and Wood, 2005, p. 242). This emphasis on body and experience also opened up a space for fat women to position themselves within mainstream feminism and as sexual agents.

One especially productive route for fat feminism of the third wave was the radical DIY riot grrrl subculture which extended far beyond its roots in the Pacific Northwest of the USA, including to the UK, Europe, South America and Australia. Fat liberation and acceptance were championed in the music – including in the names of the two most iconic bands Bikini Kill and Huggy Bear – and in the many 'zines that circulated in the riot grrrl universe' (Monem, 2007, p. 118); 'riots not diets' was an inspired mantra and 'fuck no fat chicks' was among the 'reclaimed and defanged' epithets riot grrrls scrawled on their bodies (Baumgardner and Richards, 2000, p. 78). Located within a wider politics that aimed, in the words of the 'Riot Grrrl Manifesto', to 'create revolution in our lives every single day by envisioning and creating alternatives to the bullshit christian capitalist way of doing things' (Hanna, 1991), fat positivity announced itself as creative, defiant and counter-hegemonic. The co-option of 'girl power' by apolitical pop sensations Spice Girls has been narrated as the death knell of riot grrrl, but it endures as both identification and inspiration, including for Russian feminist art collective Pussy Riot and the LadyFest feminist music and arts festival that began in London in 2001 and has since gone global: fat activism is regularly incorporated.

As for feminist scholarship on the body, its utility for fat feminism and fat studies has been acknowledged (Lupton, 2013, p. 28), but with crucial caveats. Marilyn Wann would later recall that when she first read French feminist philosophy her impression was that these feminist thinkers 'obviously did not have fat women in mind' (Erdman Farrell, 2011, p. 147). For Charlotte Cooper enduring references to the 'holy trinity' of Orbach, Chernin and Bordo two decades later as though 'feminism has dealt with the question of fat, and there is nothing more to say' marginalises the history of feminist fat activism and the contribution of fat women: not one author identifies as fat and all three have acknowledged their own eating disorders in their work (Cooper, 2010).

In the early 2000s, feminist scholars from various disciplines within which their work on fat had been marginalised pioneered Fat Studies, closely aligned to fat activism. The identification of an 'obesity' epidemic – the evidence and consequences of which are challenged directly by fat studies – has intensified feminist scholarship on fat, but differences have emerged over what constitutes the most effective 'feminist' response to the 'war on obesity' and to fat in general. In feminist journal *Signs* in 2006, Yancey, Leslie and Abel recommended moving on from the feminist view of fat as an aesthetic and moral issue to taking seriously the obesity epidemic via positive engagement with public health initiatives focused on women (Yancey et al. 2006, p. 437). Along related lines, Elspeth Probyn critiqued the strategies of fat acceptance – such as semiotic reversal and fat pride – as ineffectual political strategies that 'make an obvious point but do little to intervene in a situation where people are increasingly terrorized and seriously damaged by what they eat'; she proposed instead that feminist critique more seriously address 'the socioeconomic structures that are producing ever larger bodies' (Probyn, 2008, pp. 402–3). Fat Studies, sceptical of obesity science to begin with, also recognises the correlation of weight and class, but challenges the view that poverty causes fatness and proposes the reverse: fatness leads to poverty and fat women in particular suffer economically as a result of their size (Rothblum, 2011, p. 176). For Anna Kirkland, feminist collusion with public health discourse and campaigns renders feminism 'dangerously and naively sympathetic to public health moralism', sets it up for 'moralized interventions into women's lives' (Kirkland, 2011, p. 470) and leaves untouched the 'historical, economic and cultural context of our fat hatred' (p. 474). It is Kirkland's hope that feminist scholars draw instead on 'past disobedience to social norms about health and appearance' and to 'interrogate our ignorance, particularly about the lived experiences of women who would be targeted under anti-obesity policy' (p. 480). The history of feminist fat activism would offer a rich entry point into this project, while contemporary fat feminism that counters fatphobia by embodying and re-imagining 'fat sex' enriches feminist sexual politics generally.

Conclusion

This chapter has traced two trajectories in western feminism that are both intersecting and distinct, beginning with fat feminism or Fat Liberation which had its origins in the wider fat acceptance movement and Women's Liberation in the United States in the early 1970s. For at least the first decade, Fat Liberation was primarily directed at identifying and combatting fat oppression, particularly as directed at women. Fat Liberationists advanced their politics by mobilising as fat women with their own groups and publications and also via the wider women's movement, especially though not exclusively radical lesbian feminism. As some of the contributors to the 1983 anthology *Shadow on a Tightrope* would later recount, fat acceptance and Women's Liberation had their limits as spaces in which fat women could explore their sexuality and be positively validated by it. Fat Liberation was maintained as a goal, but to reiterate the late Heather McAllister's point, any talk of freedom was meaningless if not experienced through the body. Sex and sexuality moved to the fore of fat feminism from the 1990s, often under the auspices of a specifically 'queer', sex-positive fat feminism, exemplified by Big Burlesque, the Fat-Bottom Revue and the FaT GirL Collective.

In the 1970s and 1980s, Fat Liberation, in the US and elsewhere, was incorporated into the wider women's movement in a variety of ways, including occasional coverage in periodicals (most memorably on the cover of *Spare Rib* in 1987), at conferences and protests and primarily through the efforts of fat feminists such as Karen Stimson who promoted fat issues via the Feminist Caucus of the National Council of Women and by actively lobbying feminist publications such as *Ms*. Magazine. Compared to the coverage Susie Orbach generated for *Fat is A Feminist Issue*, however, Fat Liberation's message was muted: later fat feminist activists such as Nomy Lamm were exposed to Orbach before they were involved in Fat Liberation, though it was the latter (when she finally found it) that helped Lamm clarify why mainstream feminist treatment of fat did not speak to her. Lamm, like other fat feminist icons such as pop singer Beth Ditto of The Gossip, would later find the riot grrrl and 'queercore' scenes much more accommodating of fat bodies and of queer sexualities.

However, while third wave feminism's emphasis on embodiment and sex and its purported claims to expand feminism's constituency beyond the second-wave created new opportunities for fat-identified women to share their experiences (and as part of that, their sexualities), there have been some criticisms of the third wave generally that have since been applied to some forms of fat feminism that have emerged over the last decade. These include that fat feminism has been diluted or given way to post-feminist fat activism through an excessive emphasis on the self and sexual empowerment at the expense of collective mobilisation, radical or queer sexual agendas and/or honest accounts of the limits of fat positivity (Murray, 2005).

Further, the short histories of fat feminism and mainstream feminism narrated in this chapter may appear more teleological and converging than has actually been the case. As I have traced, the alliance of fat activism and feminism – and also fat activism and queer politics – now has a history extending over three decades, but these connections are just as likely to be rejected as embraced by some contemporary feminists – sometimes in tones and terms reminiscent of feminists who have rejected sex workers as allies: i.e. because they disapprove of their lifestyle choice.

'Fat is a Feminist Issue' endures as a slogan because it does so much necessary work in a pithy fashion: yes, feminists *must* address fat is a widely held view but beyond this consensus fragments. As a 'feminist issue' fat can manifest in many ways: the question 'is it feminist to go on a diet?' (Drews, 2007), a critique of identity politics and its limits (Crawford, 2012), and as a necessary component of feminism's commitment to intersectionality (van Amsterdam, 2013). At one end, fat stigma is recognised as having an impact on the lives of all women and is symptomatic of the unequal burden placed on women to accrue 'erotic capital' in patriarchal, capitalist societies; on the other debates about how feminism should go about addressing fat can have the effect of separating fat women from the category of 'feminist' (even if popular culture often conflates the two). The lack of historical recognition for fat feminism is one way that this separation is enacted. Sometimes Orbach's title and the book to which it's attached stand in for the history of feminism and fat, the first and the last word, resuscitated in order to demonstrate that feminism did address the issue. The historicising of fat activists such as Charlotte Cooper helps to counter historical amnesia, but the productive and creative ways that fat activists have utilised the internet to disseminate their politics, and increasingly their history, is sometimes lost on self-identified feminists who take to the internet to express reservations about fat acceptance (Hall, 2014).

Finally, as the examples catalogued here have demonstrated, fat feminists and fat feminism have addressed sex and sexuality in ways that have deepened or can advance feminist and queer sexual politics more generally. In challenging normative representations and discourses of sexual appeal, desire and practice, fat activists have also taken to task heteronormativity, 'look-ism', thin privilege, able-bodiness and sexist stereotypes that hypersexualise fat women and/or cast them as non-sexual. Their efforts have not been in vain – research has demonstrated, for instance, that the rise of fat pride has had positive effects on self-image and the sex lives of fat women (Gailey, 2012) – and are ongoing, as the possibilities of 'fat sex' are now central to fat feminism.

References

Baumgardner, Jennifer and Richards, Amy, 2000, *Manifesta: Young Women, Feminism and the Future*, Farrar, Straus and Giroux, New York.

Bean, Linda and Duguid, Beverley, 1989, 'Body Consciousness', *Spare Rib: A Women's Liberation Magazine*, No. 182, September, pp. 20–21.

Bordo, Susan, 2003, *Unbearable Weight: Feminism, Western Culture, and the Body*, University of California Press, Berkeley and Los Angeles, Tenth Anniversary edition, originally published 1993.

Chrisler, Joan C., 2012, '"Why Can't You Control Yourself": Fat *Should Be* a Feminist Issue', *Sex Roles*, Vol. 66, pp. 608–616.

Cooper, Charlotte, 2010, 'Fat is a Feminist Issue, but whose feminism?', *The Scavenger*, 11 September at: http://www.thescavenger.net/feminism-a-pop-culture-sp-9560/feminism-a-pop-culture/428-fat-is-a-feminist-issue-but-whose-feminism-90645.html.

Cooper, Charlotte, 2011, *A Queer and Trans Fat Activist Timeline*, http://obesitytimebomb.blogspot.com/p/queer-and-trans-fat-activist-timeline.html.

Cooper, Charlotte, 2012, 'A Queer and Trans Fat Activist Timeline: Queering Fat Activist Nationality and Cultural Imperialism', *Fat Studies: An Interdisciplinary Journal of Body Weight and Society*, 1:1, 61–74.

Cooper, Charlotte, 2013, 'Shadow on a Tightrope: the book that made me fat' 8 November 2013 http://obesitytimebomb.blogspot.co.uk/2013/11/shadow-on-tightrope-book-that-made-me.html. Accessed 21 January.

Crawford, Anwyn, 2012, 'Fat, privilege and resistance', *Overland*, Issue 28, http://overland.org.au/previous-issues/issue-208/feature-anwyn-crawford/.

Diamond, Nicky, 1985, 'Thin is the Feminist Issue', *Feminist Review*, No. 19, Spring, pp. 45–64.

Dickenson, Joan, 1983, 'Some thoughts on Fat' in Schoenfielder, L. and Wieser, B. (eds) *Shadow on a Tightrope: Writings by Women on Fat Oppression*, Aunt Lute Books, San Francisco, pp. 37–51.

Drews, Marie, 2007, 'Food: My Feminist Issue', *rhizomes*, 14, Summer, pp. 1–18, http://www.rhizomes.net/issue14/drews.html.

Dykewomon, Elena, 1983, 'Traveling Fat' in Schoenfielder, L. and Wieser, B. (eds) *Shadow on a Tightrope: Writings by Women on Fat Oppression*, Aunt Lute Books, San Francisco, pp. 144–154.

Edison, Laurie Toby and Notkin, Debbie, 1994, *Women En Large: Images of Fat Nudes*, Books in Focus, San Francisco.

Edut, Ophira (ed.) 2003 [1993], *Body Outlaws: Rewriting the Rules of Beauty and Body Image*, Seal Press, Emeryville.

Farrell, Amy Erdman, 2011, *Fat Shame: Stigma and the Fat Body in American Culture*, NYU Press, New York City.

Fishman, Sara Golda Bracha, 1998, 'Life in the Fat Underground', *Radiance: A Magazine for Large Women Online*, Winter 1998, 1–4, http://www.radiancemagazine.com/issues/1998/winter_98/fat_underground.html.

Fixmer, Natalie and Wood, Julia, 2005, 'The Personal is *Still* Political: Embodied Politics in Third Wave Feminism', *Women's Studies in Communication*, Vol. 28: No. 2, Fall, pp. 235–257.

Frater, Lara, 2013, 'Parallel Lives' 7 November 2013. http://fatchicksrule.blogs.com/fat_chicks_rule/2013/11/parallel-lives.html. Accessed 21 January.

Freedman, Estelle B, 2002, *No Turning Back: The History of Feminism and the Future of Women*, Profile Books, London.

Freespirit, Judy and Aldebaran 'Fat Liberation Manifesto' in Schoenfielder, L. and Wieser, B. (eds) *Shadow on a Tightrope: Writings by Women on Fat Oppression*, Aunt Lute Books, San Francisco, pp. 52–53.

Gailey, Jeannine A. (2012), 'Fat Shame to Fat Pride: Fat Women's Sexual and Dating Experiences', *Fat Studies: An Interdisciplinary Journal of Body Weight and Society*, 1:1, pp. 114–127.

Goode, Erich and Preissler, Joanne (1983) 'The fat admirer', *Deviant Behavior*, 4:2, pp. 175–202.

Hall, Carolyn, 2014, '6 Things I Don't Understand About the Fat Acceptance Movement', http://thoughtcatalog.com/carolyn-hall/2014/04/6-things-i-dont-understand-about-the-fat-acceptance-movement/.

Hanna, Kathleen, 1991, 'The Riot Grrrl Manifesto', *Bikini Kill* Zine 2. http://onewarart.org/riot_grrrl_manifesto.htm.

Harley, Cecilia, 2001, 'Letting Ourselves Go: Making room for the fat body in feminist scholarship' in J. Braziel and K. LeBesco (eds.) *Bodies out of Bounds: Fatness and Transgression*, University of California Press, Berkeley, pp. 60–73.

Heywood, Leslie and Drake, Jennifer (eds), 1997, *Third Wave Agenda: Being Feminist, Doing Feminism*, Minnesota University Press, Minneapolis.

Higginbotham, Anastasia, 1997, 'Women of the Year: Nomy Lamm', *Ms.* January/February, pp. 60–63.

Hutchins, Loraine, 1985, 'Review: *Shadow on a Tightrope: Writings by Women on Fat Oppression*', *off our backs*, Vol. 15, No. 3, pp. 24–25.

Hutchins, Loraine, 1988, 'Biatribe: A Feminist Bisexual Politic for Change', *off our backs*, Vol. 18, No. 2, pp. 16–18.

Hutchins, Loraine and Ka'ahumanu, Lani (eds), 1991, *Bi Any Other Name: Bisexual People Speak Out*, Alyson Books, Los Angeles.

Jenkins, Tina and Smith, Barbara, 1989, 'Fat Liberation', *Spare Rib: A Women's Liberation Magazine*, No. 182, September, pp. 14–18.

Kelly, 1983, 'The Goddess is Fat', in Schoenfielder, L. and Wieser, B. (eds) *Shadow on a Tightrope: Writings by Women on Fat Oppression,* Aunt Lute Books, San Francisco, pp. 15–21.

Kent, Le'A, 2001, 'Fighting Abjection: Representing Fat Women' in Braziel, Jana Evans and LeBesco, Kathleen (eds) *Bodies out of Bounds: Fatness and Trangression*, University of California Press, Berkeley, pp. 130–142.

Kirkland, Anna, 2011, 'The Environmental Account of Obesity: A Case for Feminist Skepticism', *Signs*, Vol. 36, No. 2, pp. 463–485.

Lamm, Nomy, 1995, 'It's a Big Fat Revolution', originally published in Findlen, Barbara (ed.) *Listen Up: Voices From The Next Feminist Generation*, Seal Press, online at: http://tehomet.net/nomy.html.

Lamm, Nomy, 1996, 'Fat Is Your Problem', *Ms.* March/April.

Lamm, Nomy, 1999, 'Fashion', *Ms.* April/May.

Lamm, Nomy, 2003, 'Fishnets, feather boas and fat', Ophira Edut (ed.) *Body Outlaws: Rewriting the rules of beauty and body image: expanded and updated second edition*, Seal Press, Emeryville, 78-87.

LeBesco, Kathleen, 2001, 'Queering Fat Bodies/Politics' in Braziel, Jana Evans and LeBesco, Kathleen (eds) *Bodies out of Bounds: Fatness and Trangression*, University of California Press, Berkeley, pp. 74–90.

Lepoff, Laurie Ann, 1983, 'Fat Politics', in Schoenfielder, L. and Wieser, B. (eds) *Shadow on a Tightrope: Writings by Women on Fat Oppression*, Aunt Lute Books, San Francisco, pp. 204–209 (originally published May 1975).

Lupton, Deborah, 2013, *Fat*, London and New York, Routledge.

Mabel-Lois, Lynn and Aldebaran, 1983, 'Fat Women and Women's Fear of Fat', in Schoenfielder, L. and Wieser, B. (eds) *Shadow on a Tightrope: Writings by Women on Fat Oppression*, Aunt Lute Books, San Francisco, pp. 53–57.

Mayer, Vivian F. 1983, 'Foreword' in Schoenfielder, L. and Wieser, B. (eds) *Shadow on a Tightrope: Writings by Women on Fat Oppression*, Aunt Lute Books, San Francisco, pp. ix-xxi.

McAllister, Heather, 2009, 'Embodying Fat Liberation' in Rothblum, Esther and Solovay, Sondra (eds), *The Fat Studies Reader*, New York University Press, New York, pp. 305–311.

McCarthy, Allison, 2012, 'The Politics of Fat: We Have to Keep Struggling to Liberate ourselves from Self-Hatred', www.alternet.org, April 4 at: http://www.alternet.org/story/154850/the_politics_of_fat%3A_we_have_to_keep_struggling_to_liberate_ourselves_from_self-hatred.

McRobbie, Angela, 2009, *The Aftermath of Feminism: gender, culture and social change*, Sage, London.

Monem, Nadine, 2007, *Riot Grrrl: Revolution girl style now!*, Black Dog Publishing, London.

Murray, Samantha, 2005, 'Doing Politics or Selling Out? Living the Fat Body', *Women's Studies: An Inter-disciplinary Journal*, Vol. 34, No. 3–4, pp. 265–277.

Orbach, Susie, 1985, 'Response to Nicky Diamond', *Feminist Review*, Winter, pp. 119–121.

Orbach, Susie, 2006, *Fat is a Feminist Issue: The Anti-Diet Guide* (originally published 1978) and *Fat is a Feminist Issue II* (originally published 1981), Arrow Books, London.

Probyn, Elspeth, 2008, 'Silences Behind the Mantra: Critiquing Feminist Fat', *Feminism and Psychology*, Vol. 18: 3, pp. 401–404.

Rothblum, Esther D., 2011, 'Fat Studies' in J. Cawley (ed.) *The Oxford Handbook of the Social Science of Obesity*, Oxford University Press, New York, pp. 173–183.

Rothblum, Esther, 2013. '"Shadow on a Tightrope": Continuing to throw its weight around' 8 November 2013 http://www.moreofmetolove.com/blogs/entry/shadows-on-a-tightrope-continuing-to-throw-its-weight-around/. Accessed 21 January.

Saguy, Abigail and Ward, Anna, 2011, 'Coming Out as Fat: Rethinking Stigma', *Social Psychology Quarterly*, XX(X), pp. 1–23.

Schoenfielder, Lisa and Wieser, Barb, 1983, (eds) *Shadow on a Tightrope: Writings by Women on Fat Oppression*, Aunt Lute Books, San Francisco.

Scott-Jones, Karen, 1983, 'Attraction and/or Intimidation: Fat Women's Sexual Dilemmas' in Schoenfielder, L and Wieser, B. (eds) *Shadow on a Tightrope: Writings by Women on Fat Oppression*, Aunt Lute Books, San Francisco, pp. 216–222.

Snider, Stefanie, 2009, 'Fat Girls and Size Queens: Alternative Publications and the Visualising of Fat and Queer Eroto-politics in Contemporary American Culture' in Rothblum, Esther and Solovay, Sondra (eds), *The Fat Studies Reader*, New York University Press, New York, pp. 223–231.

Snider, Stefanie, 2010, 'Revisioning Fat Lesbian Subjects in Contemporary Lesbian Periodicals', *Journal of Lesbian Studies*, 14: 2–3, pp. 174–184.

Snider, Stephanie, 2012, *Women En Large: Images of Fat Nudes*, by Laurie Toby Edison and Debbie Notkin and *The Full Body Project*, by Leonard Nimoy, Natalie Angier, and Anne Wilkes Tucker [Book Review], *Fat Studies*, Vol. 1, Issue 1, 2012, pp. 130–133.

Snyder, Claire R., 2008, 'What is Third Wave Feminism: A New Directions Essay', *Signs*, Vol. 34, No. 1, Autumn, pp. 175–196.

Stearns, Peter N., 1997, *Fat History: Bodies and Beauty in the Modern West*, New York University Press, New York.

Stimson, Karen, n.d, 'Fat Feminist Herstory, 1969–1993: A Personal Memoir', archived from http://www.eskimo.com/~largesse/Archives/herstory.html.

Stimson, Karen, 2008, 'Fat Feminism: Politics and Perspective', *Largesse: The Network for Size Esteem*, archived from http://wayback.archive.org/web/20080512074722/http://www.largesse.net/feminism.html.

Taylor, Verta and Rupp, L., 1993, 'Women's Culture and Lesbian Feminist Activism: A Reconsideration of Cultural Feminism', *Signs*, Vol. 19, No. 1, pp. 32–61.

Van Amsterdam, Noortje, 2013, 'Big Fat Inequalities: An Intersectional Perspective on 'Body Size'', *European Journal of Women's Studies*, 20: 2, pp. 155–169.

Walker, Joan (1997), 'Women of the Year', Letter to *Ms.* May/ June, p. 4.

Wann, Marilyn, 1998, *Fat! So? Because you Don't Have to Apologise for your Size*, Ten Speed Press, Berkeley.

Wann, Marilyn, 2013, 'Celebrating 30 years of 'Shadow on a Tightrope' – the book that changed my life and yours!', 8 November, http://fatso.com/2013/11/146/.

Williams, Regina D., 2003 [1993] 'Conquering the fear of a fat body: the journey to myself' in Edut, Ophira (ed.) 2003 [1993], *Body Outlaws: Rewriting the Rules of Beauty and Body Image*, Seal Press, Emeryville.

Wolf, Naomi, 1991, *The Beauty Myth: How Images of Beauty are Used Against Women*, originally published 1990, Vintage, London.

Yancey, Antronette K., Joanne Leslie, Emily K. Abel, 2006, 'Obesity at the Crossroads: Feminist and Public Health Perspective', *Signs*, Vol. 31: No. 2, Winter, pp. 425–433.

Chapter 3
Human Nature: On Fat Sexual Identity and Agency

Cat Pausé

> I think I'd be grossed out if I had to watch two characters with rolls and rolls of fat kissing each other ... because I'd be grossed out if I had to watch them doing anything. To be brutally honest, even in real life, I find it aesthetically displeasing to watch a very, very fat person simply walk across a room.

In an article about the television sitcom *Mike & Molly*, Maura Kelly (2010) expressed her disgust at the idea of having to watch the fat characters engage in displays of affection. The comments on the piece demonstrated that she is not the only one to find acts of sexual expression among fat people to be gross. But agreement was not the only response Kelly's piece received. A range of responses, from the online fat community, the online feminist community, and even mainstream presses, cried out over the fat shaming and hatred contained in the article. Emily Exton (2010) at *Entertainment Weekly* suggested in her piece that not only do viewers need to get over any objection to seeing fat people be amorous on screen, but that producers of on screen material need to get over their reliance on fat jokes to tell a fat story.

Examining more recent mainstream media coverage around fat sexuality reinforces the negative perception that many, like Kelly, may have. In the *Sydney Morning Herald*, Matty Silver (2014) argues that a better sex life can be found through weight loss. Focusing in on issues of erectile dysfunction and sterility in heterosexual men, Silver suggests that fat men often find sex difficult because of their lack of stamina or lower levels of testosterone. She also highlights the low self-esteem that may plague fat men, noting that "fat in the abdominal area can make the penis look smaller than it really is, which doesn't help self-esteem." An article from CNN (2014) promotes a new book, *XL love: How the obesity crisis is complicating American's love life*. The author of the book, Sarah Varney, suggests that fatness has a "chilling effect on sexual relationships, from physical barriers to intimacy to attitudinal shifts with weight gain and even loss." The article frames the discussion around concerns of the 'obesity epidemic' and the impact it may have on the lives of fat people.

The mainstream media's representations and discussions around sex makes it clear that fat people are not considered sexually attractive, or as individuals with sexual agency. As noted by LeBesco (2004), mainstream discourses on what is sexy and how sexy is embodied usually excludes fatness and fat bodies. Murray (2004) argues this is due to heteronormative systems that construct the values and meanings surrounding sex and sexual identification. Systems such as capitalism and neoliberalism place value on discipline, conformity, and fulfilling the fantasies of the dominant subject (heterosexual men in power). Fatness, according to these systems, is not desirable or valued. The rejection of fatness as acceptable has led to fat identity being classified as a spoiled identity; one in which the bearer of the stigma (fatness) is held responsible for the stigma (Pausé, 2012). All identities are constructed, maintained, and revised through an interaction of individual's beliefs about themselves and the messages one receives from the environment. A spoiled identity, like fatness, is further complicated by the individuals' beliefs about themselves being shaped by the internalized oppression that many in marginalized populations hold. For example, fat individuals are just as likely as non-fat individuals to hold anti-fat attitudes (Schwartz, Vartanian, Nosek, and Brownell, 2006; Wang, Brownell, and Wadden, 2004). Harding (2008) illuminates this internalized oppression and how it reflects back on fat sexual identities and behaviours, "When you're a fat woman in this culture, *everyone*—from journalists you'll never meet to your own mother, sister, and best friend—works together to constantly reinforce the message that you are not good enough to be fucked" (p. 74). The negative messages integrated into a fat person's sexual identity are then unchallenged as fat people are rarely included in displays and discourses related to sex; or reinforced as the discourses and displays that do exist in mainstream sex discourses do not look favourably upon fat sex.

If fat individuals are excluded from mainstream discourses around sex, what does this mean for a fat individual who is forming and performing an identity as a sexual being? As Murray points out,

> One only has to reflect on the ways in which we speak about fatness in this historical moment in Western societies ... We talk about fatness as a major health crisis, an epidemic, a drain on resources, a symbol of the failed body, and as an aesthetic affront. We do not talk about fat and sex. (2004, p. 239).

Perhaps Murray is correct; we do not talk about fat sex as a normative part of our discourse. It is, as LeBesco (2004) suggests, excluded from constructions of normal sexuality. So how then is fat sexual activity presented? And how are fat individuals to construct positive sexual identities in a fat hating world? This piece does not intend to propose the ways in which fat individuals construct their understanding of sexuality, or themselves as sexual beings. It does, however, attempt to consider some of the narratives presented to people around what fat sexuality means and how it is embodied and performed.

Given the prevalent anti-fat attitudes in heteronormative Western cultures, it is not surprising that most of the empirical scholarship around body size and sexuality have concluded that fat individuals, especially fat women, are significantly disadvantaged in the areas of heterosexual dating and sexual activity (Regen, 1996; Tiggemann and Rothblum, 1988; Widerman and Hurst, 2008). Focus has more recently turned to examining the impact of fatness on sexual activity and behavior.

Obesity research on sexuality can be grouped into three categories based on the sample being studied: population studies, clinical studies, and weight loss studies. In population studies, where participants are pulled from a general population, no significant relationship between weight and sexual functioning and satisfaction are found with the exception of the relationship between BMI and sexual dysfunction in men. For example, Adolfsson and others (2004) sampled 4,781 men and women, aged 18–74, and determined there to be no relationship between BMI and sexual satisfaction. In clinical studies, studies where the sample has been drawn from a specific group of individuals (such as those with an existing condition), BMI was found significant in sexual functioning and satisfaction for some clinical populations (Chung, Sohn, and Park, 1999, Esposito et al., 2007), but not all (Kadioglu et al., 2010, Paranhos et al., 2009). In weight loss, studies, however, the findings are consistent. Research drawn from samples of individuals engaged in weight loss find that weight loss improves both functioning and satisfaction (Hammoud, Gibson, Hunt, Adams, Carrell, Kolotkin, and Meikle, 2009; Kolotkin, Zunker, and Østbye, 2012; Larsen, Wagner, and Heitmann, 2007). This could suggest that individuals who are unhappy with their sex lives pursue weight loss as a possible remedy; more likely it suggests that individuals who are pursuing weight loss are unhappy with their current weight and perceive improvements in all areas of life if weight loss occurs.

As noted by a review of the literature by Kolotkin, Zunker, and Østbye (2012), most of the empirical studies around fatness and sexuality in obesity research draw from samples of individuals engaged in weight loss. And the majority of the available research in this area has focused on sexual dysfunction (often measured as erectile dysfunction in men). In their conclusion, Kolotkin, Zunker, and Østbye (2012) call for a wider understanding of sexual functioning and satisfaction in the literature.

Not surprisingly, the tenor of work in obesity research is negative; assuming from the start that being fat is negative and thus impacts negatively on sexuality. For example, several studies (Kolotkin et al., 2006, Kolotkin et al., 2008) in this area assess sexual functioning and satisfaction using the Impact of Weight on Quality of Life (IWQOL) questionnaire. The IWQOL is a 74-item survey, assessing the "perceived effect of weight on quality of life in eight key areas—health, social/interpersonal life, work, mobility, self-esteem, sexual life, activities of daily living, and comfort with food" (Kolotkin, Head, and Brookhart, 1997, p. 435). This questionnaire is grounded in a deficit view, with six questions around sexuality that inquire as to the impact of an individual's weight on: "not feeling sexually attractive," "not enjoying sexual activity," "avoidance of sexual encounters," "difficulty with sexual performance," and "not wanting to be seen undressed" (Kolotkin, Binks, Crosby, Østbye, Mitchell, and Hartley, 2008). Measures such as the IWQOL work from the position that being fat must negatively affect an individual's sex life, fitting in with the standard assumption that grounds all of obesity research: fat is bad.Slightly more positive in tone is the work surrounding heterosexual men who prefer fat sexual partners. These men are labelled Fat Admirers (FAs). FAs are likely to identify fat bodies as more attractive than non-fat bodies and regularly choose fat women as sexual partners (Swami and Tovèe, 2009). The research surrounding FAs often explores this sexual choice with a hint of disgusted curiosity while labelling it as "deviant." Who are these men who enjoy having sex with fat women? Perhaps they wish to be smothered (Murray, 2004)? Prohaska and Gailey (2009) present a piece on hogging in the *Fat Studies Reader*. Hogging is the act of straight men pursuing fat women as sexual partners, often at the bidding of friends, and for the result of satiating sexual desire in an easy manner. They argue that hogging, to the men who participate in the activity, is based on the assumption that "fat women are sexually easy and can help men out of a losing streak" (p. 158). So we have on the one hand, men who pursue fat women as sexual partners out of deviant desire, and on the other, men who pursue fat women as sexual partners to reinforce their virility.

It is not surprising that most of the scholarship on sexuality has focused on men's sexual activities, behaviors, and desires. Both within and outside academic scholarship, women have often been denied sexual agency, especially those that fall outside of heteronormative culture (Richardson, 2000). Those women routinely excluded from normative representations of sexuality (fat women, lesbian women, trans women, women of colour, etc.), are presented with the dilemma as to whether to construct their own ideas of sexuality, independent from heteronormative narratives, or to deconstruct the existing narratives and position their sexual identities as contrasting. Do they demand to be acknowledged as equal to the norm, or celebrate their differences apart from the norm (Richardson, 2000)? Or is it possible to embrace and acknowledge their unique position while refusing to accept anything less than full sexual citizenship?

Sitting outside of academic scholarship are books that are written by fat people about fat sex. Two such tomes are Rebecca Jane Weinstein's *Fat sex: The naked truth* (2012) and Virgie Tovar's *Hot and heavy: Fierce fat girls on life, love and fashion* (2012). While both books are presentations on fat sex from fat individuals, the messages of the books are strikingly different.

Fat sex: The naked truth presents itself as a book about fat sex. Weinstein's book has been crafted around narratives about sex from fat people, and people who enjoy having sex with fat people. Framing the narratives is commentary about society's perspective on fat sexuality and factoids about information relevant to understanding fat sex within our culture. Weinstein's book, unfortunately, often promotes tired ideas around fatness (suggesting that fat is the new gay, asserting that fat is the last acceptable form of prejudice, etc.) while also reinforcing many of the negative stereotypes held about fat people. The engagement of oppression Olympics has been fully deconstructed and dismissed by critical scholars (Yuval-Davis, 2012), and the narratives of unhappy fat people who vehemently wish to change their bodies (and therefore, their lives) add nothing new to the cultural understanding of fat sexual lives. As Addison (2013) in her review in *Fat Studies: An interdisciplinary journal of body weight and society* notes, "The sex in *Fat Sex* is often not very sexy" (p. 108). Addison highlights the tensions between storytelling and often poorly applied commentary that result in an awkward read. Overall, the reader of *Fat sex* may find themselves wishing that more of the personal stories had been included in the manuscript; the individual voices of fat individuals talking about their sex lives is often muted.

A very different telling of fat sexual lives may be found in Virgie Tovar's (2012) edited collection, *Hot and heavy: Fierce fat girls on life, love and fashion*. In this collection, 31 fat women share their personal stories of rejecting cultural constructions of fat shame and hatred and embracing their inner fierceness. Not all of the stories include sexuality, but many of them highlight sexual acts and identities as important part of their fat lives. All of the narratives in Tovar's text are stories of redemption. The writers share stories of embracing sexuality, encouraging others to embrace their own sexual pleasure in their fat bodies, and finding pride in oneself through sexual identity and agency. These narratives, while more positive than those presented in *Fat Sex*, are still often problematic. Many of the stories presented rely on patriarchal assertions that a women's worth is based in her ability to be desirable to others (specifically, heterosexual men). Averill (2014) notes in her review of the book that finding one's fierceness in the male gaze denies women sexual agency and "perpetuates a world in which women only exist as powerful when they are beauty objects" (p. 66). As represented by the many of the essays in Tovar's collection, this is not an uncommon experience. The focus for heterosexual fat women in mainstream media images is usually on validating their sexual desirability (Kyrölä, 2014). In contrast, representations of heterosexual fat men in media (think *Shallow Hal* or *The Nutty Professor*) focus on validating their sexual desires. Kyrölä notes that this is not an unusual gender split; it is simply yet another example of the male gaze (Mulvey, 1975).

Alongside the scholarship from obesity research, and collections published by fat individuals, are the writings of fat women who embrace their bodies and enjoy the pleasure they may take from them. Much of this work is presented in a self-help fashion; written both to express the individual's own pleasure in sexuality, but also as a means of assisting others in experiencing a more satisfying sex life.

One of the best known self-help books for fat people is *Big big love* by Hanne Blank (2000, 2011). Blank's reputation as a producer of positive fat sex materials began with her short lived zine, *Zaftig!* and the subsequent publication of *Zaftig: Well-rounded erotica* (2001). The book is a practical, instructional, and dare it be said, inspirational, guide on relationships and sexual activity for fat individuals and their partner(s). The revised text is heavily influenced by the growing fat activism movement, the emergence of fat studies within academia, and the advancement of sexual politics in the decade since the original release. Also included in the 2011 edition is information drawn from the Big Big Love Survey, collected by Blank in 2010 from over 700 participants. Blank weaves the information shared by participants into the revised edition, often using survey material to illustrate her arguments.

Blank's sex positive tome covers a range of sexual topics, including physical accommodations with bellies for better sex, and gentle advice on how to negotiate through the internalized fat hatred that often rears to the surface when nakedness and pleasure are involved. Blank also presents discussions of ethics in fax sex, taking a considered approach to addressing Fat Admirers in the segment, "How not to be an asshole." Concerns around how to not be an asshole, as Blank presents it, are common for those interested in engaging in fat positive sex with a fat partner. This has been addressed by others, including Bevin Branlandingham in her work on being an ally to a fat lover and Marianne Kirby in her guide to sexy fun for fatties.

In February 2013, Bevin Branlandingham hosted 'Fat Sex Week' on her blog, *The Queer Fat Femme Guide to Life*.[1] Through the expanded week, Bevin shared posts about fat sex, including playlists to get the reader in the mood, reviews of fat sex tools such as the Plus Size Liberator Wedge, and suggestions for books written to help people have hot fat sex. In one post, Bevin (2013) considers ways to be a good ally to a fat lover. She writes, "All humans are worthy of sexual adoration exactly as they are," and suggests that allies of fat lovers need to banish fatphobic rhetoric from their lexicon.

In her piece, 'How to have sex while fat: A short guide to sexy fun for fatties and people who f#&@ them,' Marianne Kirby (2013) suggests that being fat sex positive is not advocating that all people must have sex with fat people. She suggests that the taboo that surrounds fat sex (and turns it into a fetish) often makes it difficult for fat people to develop sexual identity and enjoy

1 Find the 'Fat Sex Week Table of Contents' on *The Queer Fat Femme Guide to Life* at http://queerfatfemme.com/tag/fat-sex-week/.

sexual activity. She suggests some simple guidelines for navigating through the taboo, the internalization fat hatred, and the myth that fat people are not sexual beings. First, Marianne proposes, avoid sexual partners who make you feel bad about your body. Other suggestions include being communicative with your partner about what you like and what you don't, and being willing to try new things. (Those three suggestions are probably useful for people of any size.) Suggestions for those interested in having sex with a fat person include ensuring that the attraction is not all about the fat, and checking in with what your partner likes (and doesn't like), while trying out a variety of positions and tools that may help make each other comfortable. Kirby, for example, cautions, "Don't be afraid of touching your fat lover's body. Figure out what you love about the experience. Never, ever say, 'I never thought I could enjoy sex with a fat person.'" While Branlandingham and Kirby share advice for both fat individuals and their partners, others have focused solely on providing useful information for fat people. Asserting that fat people are often denied sexual agency, Kitty Stryker takes to her blog to present tips and tricks for hot fat sex. She begins by exploring a variety of ways to set the mood; Stryker suggests that many fat people struggle with feeling sexy. "We're not encouraged to love our jiggly bits," she writes. Common mood setters are suggested, including candles, massage, blindfolds, and lotions. She also presents a selection of body positive pornography, highlighting ones for queer bodies. Sex pillows, toys, and body accommodating positions are also included in her post. The inclusion of tools and techniques is common in pieces about fat sex, and suggests a market for such items. Perhaps this is one way that fat sex will become more mainstream, as capitalistic systems will embrace the opportunity to provide desirable goods to individuals looking to facilitate fat sex. Less common is pictorial how-to material, as found in the work by msvaginascience.

In "Fat sex: What everyone wants to know but is afraid to ask" msvaginascience introduces herself as a fat woman who has enjoyable sex with partners who are usually smaller than she is. Her biggest piece of advice is that fat women need to "overcome the idea that your partner doesn't know how fat you are." She unpacks this by assuring that sexual partners are aware of your body size, regardless of whether the lights are off and what position(s) you may contort your body into. Relax, she chides, they are having sex with you because they are attracted to you and want to experience your body just as it is! She then dives into advice around tools and tricks to help; echoing the self-help suggestions covered by the pieces above. For a marked difference though, msvaginascience spends most of the piece exploring different sexual positions and how they can work for fat bodies. These pieces are accompanied by pictorial illustration of her (clothed) fat body demonstrating.

This is in no way an exhaustive accounting of the materials about fat sex that have been written by fat individuals, merely a selection of the better known offerings available. The introduction of the World Web Wide, and Web 2.0, has opened up a never ending supply of spaces for individuals of all sizes to share information (Pausé, 2014a). It has especially been taken up by individuals in marginalized groups, whose sexuality is often denied (or, at least, ignored) by mainstream media and culture.

Participation in fat positive communities, both online and off, may be one way for fat people to develop positive sexual identities. "In a culture that rarely associates fat bodies with sexuality, publicly claiming sexual agency, desire, and desirability allows fat women to take pleasure in their bodies" (p. 300), writes Asbill (2009) in her chapter on fat burlesque in the *Fat studies reader*. In her qualitative work, Asbill explores the experience of fat women participating in burlesque, and considers how this activity shapes their fat identity. Engaging in explicitly sexual performance for others allowed the women involved to "[redefine] the fat body as an object of sexual desire" (p. 300). Performance is an important part of identity, as demonstrated by the women in Asbill's work. These women were given/took permission to publicly perform as fat sexual beings, allowing themselves to develop or reinforce positive fat sexual identities. Doing so in a group allowed these women to support each other through the process. Fat positive communities provide safe spaces for individuals to construct positive fat identities; for some, they may be the only spaces in which fat positive identities may be constructed, maintained, and performed.

Gailey (2012) interviewed over 30 fat women from size/fat acceptance organizations about their romantic and sexual lives. The women in her study reported having poor body image and unsatisfactory romantic and sexual histories, illustrating that body image dissatisfaction often detracts from sexual agency in women. This changed for most, however, when these women became involved in size acceptance, and began to take pride in their fat bodies. "Women who accept their bodies, or are beginning to, not only experience freedom from the pressure to diet or change their bodies, but also a freedom to be sexual," argues Gailey (p. 124). Without body image satisfaction, it is difficult to construct positive sex identities, as Gailey found in her work. Engaging in fat positive communities allowed these women to construct fat positive sexual identities.

Is it surprising that women produce much of the fat positive sex information? Perhaps this stems from the (re)production of dominant theories of social phenomena that position women and their experiences as "inferior, deviant, or significant only in the ways they serve male interests" (Anderson, 2012). Feminist epistemologies suggest that women have historically been excluded from inquiry and epistemic authority. This may be seen as reinforced by the focus in obesity research on sexuality on sexual dysfunction, specifically, erectile dysfunction. In contrast, fat positive sex resources suggest that fat sex is enjoyable and normative. And they argue that fat people are sexual beings with sexual agency who are engaging in satisfying sex lives; a stark juxtaposition to the themes in the literature of obesity research.

As individuals increasingly produce large amounts of knowledge in the Web 2.0 age, marginalized communities are able to present their truths and suggest representations of themselves that contrast the dominant discourses (Pausé, 2014b). If, as Gailey (2012) suggests, involvement in size acceptance leads to decreased body image dissatisfaction and greater sexual agency for fat women, then perhaps turning to fat activist communities for information about sex, and drawing on sexuality scholarship from the field of Fat Studies (a field that rejects the negative assumptions associated with fatness and the fat body) will allow more fat women to construct positive fat sexual identities and exercise their sexual agency.

References

Addison, S. 2013. Where "fat" and "Sex" intersect. *Fat Studies: An Interdisciplinary Journal of Body Weight and Society*, 2 (1), 105–109.

Adolfsson, B., Elofsson, S., Rössner, S. and Undén, A. L. 2004. Are sexual dissatisfaction and sexual abuse associated with obesity? *Obesity Research*, 12, 1702–1709.

Anderson, E. 2013. Feminist epistemology and philosophy of science. In E. N. Zalta (ed.), *The Stanford Encyclopedia of Philosophy*. Retrieved from http://plato.stanford.edu/entries/feminist-social-epistemology/ (1 August 2014).

Asbill, L. (2009). "I'm allowed to be a sexual being": The distinctive social conditions of the fat burlesque stage. In E. Rothblum and S. Solovay (eds) *The fat studies reader* (pp. 299–304), New York: New York University Press.

Averill, L. I. 2014. Virgie Tovar's first glitter-filled strike in the fat revolution. Review of *Hot and heavy: Fierce fat girls on life, love and fashion*, by Virgie Tovar. *Fat Studies: An Interdisciplinary Journal of Body Weight and Society*, 3 (1), 65–67.

Blank, H. 2011. *Big big love, revised: A sex and relationships guide for people of size (and those who love them)*. Berkeley: Celestial Arts.

Blank, H. 2001. *Zaftig: Well-rounded Erotica*. San Francisco: Cleis Press.

Branlandingham, B. 2013. 7 ways to be a good ally to your fat lover. The Frisky. Retrieved from http://www.thefrisky.com/2013–02–20/7-ways-to-be-a-good-ally-to-your-fat-lover/ (1 July 2013).

Chung, W. S., Sohn, J. H., and Park, Y. Y. 1999. Is obesity an underlying factor in erectile dysfunction?. *European Urology*, 36(1), 68–70.

Esposito, K., Ciotola, M., Giugliano, F., Bisogni, C., Schisano, B., Autorino, R., Cobellis, L., De Sio, M., Colacurci, N., and Giugliano, D. 2007. Association of body weight with sexual function in women. *International Journal of Impotence Research*, 19(4), 353–357.

Exton, E. 2010. Should 'fatties' get a room? No. But it is time for TV to move beyond fat jokes. Entertainment Weekly [online]. Retrieved from http://popwatch.ew.com/2010/10/28/marie-claire-fatties-mike-and-molly/(30 April 2014).

Gailey, J. A. 2012. Fat shame to fat pride: Fat women's sexual and dating experiences. *Fat Studies: An Interdisciplinary Journal of Body Weight and Society*, 1 (1), 114–127.

Hammoud, A., Gibson, M., Hunt, S. C., Adams, T. D., Carrell, D. T., Kolotkin, R. L., and Meikle, A. W. 2009. Effect of Roux-en-Y gastric bypass surgery on the sex steroids and quality of life in obese men. *The Journal of Clinical Endocrinology & Metabolism*, 94(4), 1329–1332.

Harding, K. 2008. How do you fuck a fat woman? In J. Friedman and J. Valenti, *Yes means yes! Visions of female sexual power & a world without rape* (pp. 67–76). Berkeley: Seal Press.

Kadioglu, P., Yetkin, D. O., Sanli, O., Yalin, A. S., Onem, K., and Kadioglu, A. 2010. Obesity might not be a risk factor for female sexual dysfunction. *BJU International*, 106(9), 1357–1361.

Kaukua, J., Pekkarinen, T., Sane, T., and Mustajoki, P. 2012. Sex hormones and sexual function in obese men losing weight. *Obesity Research*, 11 (6), 689–694.

Kelly, M. 2010. Should fatties get a room? (Even on TV)? Marie Claire [online]. Retrieved from http://www.marieclaire.com/sex-love/dating-blog/overweight-couples-on-television (29 April 2014).

Kirby, M. 2013. How to have sex while fat: A short guide to sexy fun for fatties and people who f#&@ them. xoJane [online]. Retrieved from http://www.xojane.com/sex/sex-with-a-fat-person (21 March 2013).

Kolotkin, R. L., Zunker, C., and Østbye, T. 2012. Sexual functioning and obesity: A review. *Obesity*, 20 (12), 2325–2333.

Kolotkin, R. L., Binks, M., Crosby, R. D., Østbye, T., Mitchell, J. E., and Hartley, G. 2008. Improvements in sexual quality of life after moderate weight loss. *International Journal of Impotence Research*, 20 (5), 487–492.

Kolotkin, R. L., Binks, M., Crosby, R. D., Østbye, T., Gress, R. E., and Adams, T. D. 2006. Obesity and sexual quality of life. *Obesity*, 14(3), 472–479.

Kyrölä, K. (2014). *The weight of images: Affect, body image and fat in the media.* Farnham: Ashgate.

Larsen, S. H., Wagner, G., and Heitmann, B. L. 2007. Sexual function and obesity. *International Journal of Obesity*, 31, 1189–1198.

LeBesco, K. (2004). *Revolting bodies? The struggle to redefine fat identity*. Amherst: University of Massachusetts Press.

LeTrent, S. 2014. 'XL love': How fat is affecting our sex lives. CNN [online]. Retrieved from http://edition.cnn.com/2014/07/22/living/obesity-sex-xl-love-relate/ (10 August 2014).

Msvaginascience. 2012. Fat sex: What everyone wants to know but is afraid to ask. Persephone Magazine. Retrieved from http://persephonemagazine.com/2012/03/fat-sex-what-everyone-wants-to-know-but-is-afraid-to-ask/ (1 July 2013).

Mulvey, L. 1975. Visual pleasure and narrative cinema. *Screen*, 16 (3), 6–18.

Murray, S. 2004. Locating aesthetics: Sexing the fat woman. *Social Semiotics*, 14, 237–247.

Paranhos, M., Antunes, A., Andrade, E., Freire, G., and Srougi, M. 2009. The prevalence of erectile dysfunction among Brazilian men screened for prostate cancer. *BJU International*, 104(8), 1130–1133.

Pausé, C. J. 2014a. Express yourself: Fat activism. In R. Chastain (ed.), *The politics of size: Perspectives from the fat-acceptance movement* (pp. 1-8). Santa Barbara: Praeger Publishing.

Pausé, C. J. 2014b. Causing a commotion: Queering fatness in cyberspace. In C. Pausé, J. Wykes, and S. Murray (eds) *Queering fat embodiment* (pp. 75-88). London: Ashgate.

Pausé, C. J. 2012. Live to tell: Coming out as fat. *Somatechnics*, 2 (1), 42–56.

Prohaska, A. and Gailey, J. 2009. Fat women as "easy targets": Achieving masculinity through hogging. In E. Rothblum and S. Solovay (eds) *The fat studies reader* (pp. 158–166), New York: New York University Press.

Ratliff, J. 2013. Drawing on burlesque: Excessive display and fat desire in the work of Cristina Vela. *Fat Studies: An Interdisciplinary Journal of Body Weight and Society*, 2 (2), 118–131.

Regan, P. C. 1996. Sexual outcasts: The perceived impact of body weight and gender on sexuality. *Journal of Applied Social Psychology*, 26, 1803–1815.

Richardson, D. 2000. Claiming citizenship? Sexuality, citizenship and lesbian/feminist theory. *Sexualities*, 3 (2), 255–272.

Schwartz, M. B., Vartanian, L. R., Nosek, B. A., and Brownell, K. D. 2006. The influence of one's own body weight on implicit and explicit anti-fat bias. *Obesity*, 14 (3), 440–447.

Silver, M. 2014. Lose weight for better sex. The Sydney Morning Herald [online]. Retrieved from http://www.smh.com.au/lifestyle/diet-and-fitness/lose-weight-for-better-sex-20140721-zv6vv.html (5 August 2014).

Stryker. K. 2011. Fuck me, I'm fat: A hot guide to fat sex. Kitty Stryker: PurrVersatility [Weblog]. Retrieved from http://kittystryker.com/2011/06/fuck-me-im-fat-a-hot-guide-to-fat-sex/ (1 July 2013).

Swami, V. and Tovèe, M. J. 2009. Big beautiful women: The body size preferences of male fat admirers. *Journal of Sex Research*, 46, 89–96.

Tiggemann, M., and Rothblum, E. 1988. Gender differences in social consequences of perceived overweight in the United States and Australia. *Sex Roles*, 18, 75–86.

Tovar, V. (ed.) 2012. *Hot and heavy: Fierce fat girls on life, love and fashion.* Berkeley: Seal Press.

Wang, S. S., Brownell, K. D., and Wadden, T. A. 2004. The influence of the stigma of obesity on overweight individuals. *International Journal of Obesity*, 28, 1333–1337.

Weinsten, R. J. 2012. *Fat sex: The naked truth.* Self-published: CreateSpace Independent Publishing Platform.

Widerman, M. W. and Hurst, S. R. 2008. Body size, physical attractiveness, and body image among young adult women: Relationships to sexual experience and sexual esteem. *Journal of Sex Research*, 35, 272–281.

Yuval-Davis, N. 2012. Dialogical epistemology— An intersectional resistance to the "Oppression Olympics." *Gender & Society*, 26 (1), 46–54.

Fat Gender Politics

Chapter 4
Transforming the Looking-Glass: Fat Women's Sexual Empowerment through Body Acceptance

Jeannine A. Gailey

Introduction

In Western societies, women are under tremendous pressure to conform to an increasingly narrow standard of beauty, including engaging in beauty rituals that appeal to the male gaze. Currently, thinness is equated with beauty and vitality while fatness is considered repulsive and an indication of ill health (Hesse-Biber, 2007). Fat persons are frequently regarded as lazy and gluttonous partly because the popular discourse stresses that fat is the result of overeating and lack of exercise. In other words, fat persons are "at fault" for their size and can change their predicament (lose weight) if they expend more calories than they consume. Women who are not conventionally attractive (thin) are frequently chastised, discriminated against, and labeled deviant. For instance, women of size are routinely paid less, less likely to be hired, less likely to marry (Ernsberger, 2009), and are sometimes mistreated in public by strangers who shout sizeist epithets or stare disapprovingly (Gailey, 2014). Research has found that women's self-worth is also frequently tied to their own perception of attractiveness (Patrick, Neighbors, and Knee, 2004), and since the dominant discourse stresses that fat is unattractive, it is not surprising that many women of size have embodied that viewpoint (Gailey, 2014).

Large women are often held—paradoxically—at opposing ends of a sexual spectrum, from nonsexual to sexually insatiable and desperate (Murray, 2004; Prohaska and Gailey, 2009; Boero, 2012). These are obviously stereotypes, but there is limited scholarly literature[1] that focuses specifically on fat women's sexual experiences (for exceptions, see Murray, 2004; Gailey, 2012; Satinsky et al., 2013;

1 There are some non-academic works that have focused on fat sex such as Hanne Blank's *Big Big Love* and Rebecca Weinstein's *Fat Sex*.

Gailey, 2014). Most of the research has concentrated on perceivers' opinions about fat persons' sexuality (Regan, 1996; Harris, 1990), or men's exploitative sexual experiences with fat women as "hoggers"[2] (Gailey and Prohaska, 2006) or fat admirers (Goode and Preissler, 1983; Swami and Tovèe, 2009).

This chapter contributes to the literature by focusing on several themes that emerged from in-depth interviews with 74 North American fat women about their sexual and dating experiences. More specifically, I highlight the multiple ways in which these women have learned to accept their bodies. These data indicate that the process of learning to embrace one's size tends to facilitate sexual empowerment and satisfaction. Some of the paths that led to greater body acceptance involved the discovery of size acceptance ideology,[3] online dating, experimentation and participation in alternative sexual lifestyles, involvement in body positive activities, loving and adoring partners, and growing older.

Fat Women and Sexuality

In popular culture, representations of fat women as sexual are rare. This is likely because body size is connected to the heteronormative system of meaning and value that establishes what it means to be masculine and feminine (Murray 2004). In the Western world, the gender order is configured such that hegemonic masculinity provides the parameters for the way "real" men should comport themselves and the type of women they should be attracted to, date, or marry (Connell, 1987). Women are expected to meet the normative standards of beauty (thinness) or emphasized femininity (Connell, 1987). Moreover, emphasized femininity perpetuates hegemonic masculinity and heteronormativity. Fat bodies are not typically considered attractive because fat "symbolizes domination or resistance to idealized femininity and overconsumption" (Gailey, 2012, p. 116). In some respects, fat women's bodies demonstrate characteristics associated with both masculinity and femininity. Fat is masculine because of the physical space it requires and it is extraordinarily feminine because it is soft and curvy (Lupton, 2012; Gailey, 2014).

Fat women are considered deviant, in part, because they fail to meet the prescribed Western standards of emphasized femininity. They are stereotyped as out-of-control and unmotivated to change or 'fix' their bodies. They are also

2 Hogging is a practice where men, usually college-aged, try to have a sexual encounter with a woman they deem fat or ugly for the purpose of a competition among one another or because they claim to be "hard up" (Gailey and Prohaska, 2006).

3 In this chapter, I do not discuss the direct impact the size acceptance movement has had on 26 of the women in this sample because I focus on that in a previously published manuscript (Gailey, 2012).

assumed to be incapable of managing their desires and, in turn, are sexually desperate (Prohaska and Gailey, 2009). Fat is perceived as a threat to the heteronormative system because: a) men who are attracted to fat women have failed to embody hegemonic masculinity, and b) fat women who easily find and pursue partners subvert the conventional beauty norms and feminine discourse.

Transformation of the Looking-Glass: Stigma, Embodiment, and Self-Acceptance

In addition to being considered unattractive, the fat body is radically stigmatized. Therefore, it is not surprising that many fat persons internalize fat hatred (Gailey, 2014). Gailey (2014) argues that Waskul and Vannini's (2006) concept of the 'looking glass body'—an extension Cooley's (1902) concept of the 'looking-glass self'—provides one explanation for how this happens. The 'looking-glass self' is a process where one sees him or herself from the imaginary perspective of others. The 'looking glass body' functions similarly in that we see our bodies from the perspective of others, or what we imagine others see. For instance, when we look at others' bodies we interpret what we observe and others imagine what we may be seeing and feeling—completing the reflection of the looking-glass (Waskul and Vannini, 2006, p. 5).

In Western cultures, fat is not just a failure of the body; it is also viewed as a failure of the person or an abomination of the body (Goffman, 1963). People who are fat are often characterized as lazy, irresponsible, and ignorant. Because the stigma associated with fatness is so great, it is extraordinarily difficult to accept that one is fat. Gailey (2014) found that a common phrase repeated by women she interviewed was, 'I'm not that,' by which they meant to distance themselves from the stereotypes society holds about fat people. Many interviewees embodied fat hatred. They hated other fat people and they hated themselves, but at the same time they felt like they could separate who they *really* are from other fat people.

The embodied subject is profoundly marked by its environment, including its interactions with others. However, this does not mean that the body is a blank slate upon which political discourses are inscribed. Rather, the body is understood as an active, dynamic site, one that always contains the possibility of resistance, and one that takes up the elements of its surroundings in sometimes surprising ways. If bodies are capable of resisting power dynamics, they are also capable of perpetuating them: embodied subjects, then, are deeply enmeshed in social and political forces (Turner, 1996).

To embody fat is a tremendous accomplishment because it means generally overcoming the negative messages and stereotypes propagated in the culture—a transformation of the looking-glass. Gailey's (2012) study found that women who embodied fat pride—that is, they began to embrace their fat body—as a result of subscribing to or participating in the size acceptance movement reported higher levels of sexual satisfaction. The path toward self-acceptance, for some, was made easier from learning about the Health at Every Size (HAES®)[4] ideology and other size acceptance messages. However, this chapter indicates that there are additional ways in which bodily acceptance comes about. For example, online dating, involvement in the alternative lifestyle community, engagement in activities like exercise or dance that help one become more connected to their body and its limits and strengths, through loving and adoring partners, and getting older. To build on Gailey's (2012) previous work, this chapter highlights those other paths to bodily acceptance that does not necessarily include the adoption of the size acceptance movement's ideology (see also Gailey, 2014).

The Present Study

As part of a larger study, I conducted two sets of in-depth, semi-structured interviews with 74 fat North American women between 2009 and 2012 (see also Gailey, 2014). I recruited the first 36 women from various size acceptance listservs, social networking groups, and blogs.[5] I recruited the remaining 38 from Facebook posts, Craigslist personals, Yahoo! weight loss groups, and local bariatric surgery groups. The major difference between the two samples was that the women in the former group were slightly more accepting of their bodies, a result they attributed to reading the size acceptance literature and blogs. Nevertheless, it was clear that the first sample had not completely embodied their size: the overwhelming majority indicated that if there were a magic pill that would make them thin that they would take it. Moreover, both samples of women described their feelings about their bodies in remarkably similar terms. For instance, most expressed that it is incredibly difficult to completely accept one's (fat) body in a culture that is extraordinarily fatphobic.

4 Health at Every Size (HAES)® stresses accepting one's body regardless of weight or ability and includes an emphasis on the importance of movement and exercise for enjoyment and physical pleasure, listening to one's internal bodily cues, and eating for nourishment. HAES does not encourage weight loss or dieting and intentionally separates weight from health (Bacon, 2010).

5 These women all read or subscribed to size acceptance listservs, blogs, or social networking groups. Five of the 36 identified as size acceptance activists, eight were slightly more involved through research or art, but most (63 percent) indicated that their involvement was limited to reading blogs, newsletters, and other online posts or emails.

The inclusion criteria for both studies were the same: women over 18 with a BMI greater than or equal to 30 ("obese"). I used BMI for the inclusion criteria because I did not want to make subjective decisions about who was "large enough" to participate. I recognize the problems associated with BMI as an indicator of body size, but for the purposes of the present study it was useful to provide a cut-off and is used for descriptive purposes only.

The final sample consisted of 74 North American women whose ages ranged from 19–62. Six identified as African American, five identified as Latina (Dominican, Mexican, Brazilian), one as mixed ethnicity Latina (Mexican and Brazilian), one Native American, one Gambian West African, and 60 as Caucasian, two of whom are Canadian. Nine women identified as bisexual and three as exclusively lesbian, although all three previously had relationships with men. One woman had taken a celibacy vow in her forties and another was a self-described virgin. Otherwise, the sample's sexual experiences ranged from only a couple of partners to well over 100.

The interviews consisted of open-ended questions and took place either over the phone or in person (when location allowed). There were no distinguishable differences between the phone and in person interviews, except that I obviously could not see the body language of those I spoke with on the phone. The interviews ranged from 45 minutes to four and a half hours with the average interview lasting two hours and 25 minutes.

I employed grounded theory to analyze these data. Grounded theory is an analytic technique where the researcher codes the data as it is collected so that she can utilize theoretical sampling, a process whereby the researcher seeks information on themes that arise from the subsequent participants (Charmaz and Mitchell, 2001). As patterns and themes emerged from the interviews additional questions were asked in the subsequent interviews to further tease out the distinctions until a theoretical model developed and a point of saturation was achieved, meaning the data yielded no new findings (Glaser and Strauss, 1967). In the following section, I discuss the main themes that emerged with regard to meeting partners, embracing one's body, and how that impacted sexual satisfaction.

Findings

The themes that emerged from these interviews revealed several things about the ways in which women of size negotiate a culture that tends to place them on opposite ends of a sexual spectrum—nonsexual to hypersexual. First, most participants, except those who were married and a handful who felt it was too impersonal, at some point relied on the Internet to meet partners. Second, participants tended to find ways to overcome negative stereotypes and self-hatred. Online dating seemed to help facilitate bodily acceptance and sexual empowerment partly because interviewees realized that there are people who are genuinely attracted to larger women. They also reported that this new avenue for meeting partners allowed them to explore their sexuality, including discovering their preferences and needs during sex. In addition to meeting partners online, alternative sexual lifestyles, body positive activities, adoring partners, and simply growing older all helped participants reach greater bodily acceptance. The following paths toward self-acceptance and sexual empowerment are not mutually exclusive, but often overlapped as the reflection in the looking-glass changed.

The Internet Makes it Easy

Roughly 25 million people in the U.S. (Finkel et al., 2012) turn to the Internet to meet partners for both long-term relationships and casual encounters. Given the widespread usage of the Internet to meet potential partners, it is not surprising that 60 percent of the present sample met partners on dating websites, big beautiful women (BBW) online groups, or Craigslist. These women indicated that the Internet provided them with greater options for meeting partners because they could "put it all out there," meaning that they could be "up front" about being fat and if potential suitors were not interested, they did not have to communicate with them. Dating sites and online BBW groups created a space to meet people who are genuinely attracted to larger women. In the quotes below, Corina[6] and Mary explain why online dating is so appealing.

> I was discussing this with a slim friend because I think her experience of dating was so wildly different, because she, you know, could pick guys up in bars. She was meeting people at parties, and you know, I've never had that experience, and so when I'm explaining to her that online dating works for me, like I just don't think she could even see that the world she operated in as a college kid—or now—it's so wildly different from the world I'm operating in. (Corina, 41, single)

> I was lucky that the Internet thing kind of came to be during the years that I was sequestered in my relationship with Tim. And the Internet thing for a person like me makes it very easy, because you can kind of put everything out there. You're not in the kind of situation where somebody is like picking you out in a room, or you're picking them out in a room, and you have to decide whether or not it's okay. Like I could pretty much lay my cards on the table and be like yeah, I'm a fat person. (Mary, 40, cohabitating)

---

6 All names are pseudonyms to ensure anonymity of the participants.

Both Corina and Mary revealed that they thought the Internet made it easier for them as large women to meet partners, especially because they felt like they do not have the same opportunities as "thin" women. Both mentioned the difficulties trying to meet partners at a bar or in person. Their bodies marked them as "not dateable" or undesirable in conventional settings because of the stigma associated with fat, but online there is a much larger pool of prospective partners. Even men who are "fat admirers" (men who prefer fat women) might he hesitant to flirt with a woman of size in public because of the fear of a "courtesy stigma"—being stigmatized for associating with a stigmatized person or group (Goffman, 1963)—whereas online they are shielded from the judgmental gaze of their peers. Goode and Preissler's (1983) research on "fat admirers" found that most are in the closet because of the potential 'courtesy stigma' and because it is seen as a failure of hegemonic masculinity, unless the man is doing it for sport or "hogging" (Gailey and Prohaska, 2006), a practice where men intentionally seek out women they deem fat for sex only to later humiliate them.

However, not everyone felt that online dating was rewarding or the best place to meet people. Several women talked about feeling like many of the men on online dating sites were preying on large women and others indicated that the men they met had different expectations than they did—i.e., the men expected sex and the women did not. This seemed to be a more common experience for those using free sites, BBW groups, and Craigslist.

> I—sexually was with a couple of different women at one point, not at the same time, at different times, and I was also—I actually used to go to sex parties where there were guys that liked big beautiful women. It was from a Yahoo group, actually, that I connected with it, and you know, I did that, and I just kind of felt used and disappointed again. (Janet, 36, single)

Despite the fact that some women did not have positive experiences with online dating, most did and the overwhelming majority who are single continue to use online dating as a method to meet potential partners.

Online dating opened up a world of possibilities that many women indicated was not previously available to them. They shared with me that they could more easily experiment sexually with what they liked and did not like and pick and choose among a variety of potential partners. Online dating tended to provide the women with a confidence boost when they realized that there are people who are attracted to fat women who are not all, as one interviewee stated, "losers." The experience of online dating was, for the most part, sexually empowering because it facilitated confidence, myriad experiences, and sexual growth. Corina, Mary, and numerous other interviewees felt that online dating was safer for fat women because they can "put it all out there" and avoid possible rejection from people who are not attracted to fat women.

Alternative Sexual Lifestyles

Sixteen women engaged in alternative sexual lifestyles, including participation in BDSM (bondage, discipline, sadomasochism), open relationships, polyamory (more than one lover and/or relationship), and group or public sex. Seven women were actively involved in BDSM and 10 experimented with various forms of BDSM, eight women identified as currently or previously involved in polyamorous or open relationships, and nine women had engaged in public or group sex (see also Gailey, forthcoming). There is some overlap in these categories. Three women had engaged in all three of these alternative sexual lifestyles and three engaged in two of them. Just as being involved in the size acceptance community had a positive impact on some respondents' body image and sexual expressiveness (Gailey, 2012), involvement in an alternative lifestyle relationship or finding the kink community had similar effects.

> And it was really interesting, 'cause I kind of opened up to him about being a dom[inant], because he's a natural dom[inant], I realized, in our relationship. And I was a natural submissive. And I just kind of said, 'Would you be interested?' And, actually, he was the first one I had actually kind of approached about doing anal and getting into it. And, so we kind of, just our tastes and experimentation continues to grow. (Sally, 46, divorced)

Sally has found that involvement in a dominant and submissive relationship has helped her come to accept her body and truly enjoy sex. She explained to me that communication is of the utmost importance in a BDSM relationship and that has helped her learn to be open about her wants and desires, which has led to increased confidence and bodily acceptance. She told me that over the course of her life she has had numerous partners because she was looking for approval from men or some sort of affirmation that she was pretty enough or at least worthy of men's attention—her current relationship, she said, has finally stopped that.

Other women who are also involved in BDSM relationships mentioned strikingly similar unintended consequences. Veronica said that she used to think that men were not attracted to her and that she used to worry about having sex with someone new because of her body, but since she started participating in BDSM it has changed the way she sees her body and her sexual satisfaction to the point where she prefers BDSM to "vanilla" sex.

> I prefer—I think it's more interesting that way. It's like I can have normal sex with anybody. I want it to be different. Because there is so much more, like you get the adrenaline rush and it's just so much more intense. (Veronica, 28, married)

Veronica and her husband engage in BDSM play, but they are also in an open relationship and Veronica has a boyfriend with whom she plays with too. She met her boyfriend through a BBW group and told me that she feels so much prettier now and is not nearly as self-conscious as she was prior to living an alternative sexual lifestyle.

Several of the participants thought that the BDSM community was more accepting of fat bodies. Newmahr's (2011) ethnographic work in a BDSM community also revealed that a number of the members, both men and women, were "obese"; however, Newmahr writes that weight was not a significant part of the discourse. Newmahr explained it was not that fatness was desired, but it was also not stigmatized—it ceased to be a social marker. In this particular community, and others as described by my participants, the BDSM community was a safe place where they were not marginalized for their body size.

It is not just in the BDSM community where one finds sexual empowerment through alternative lifestyles. Several women spoke about their involvement in swinger's parties and group sex events and how freeing it became, once they found the right group. Tamara, 34 and married, made it very clear to me that if she wanted to attend a group sex event or meet a new partner that she had to use groups that cater to women of size because she is at the higher end of the weight spectrum (500 pounds). When Tamara discovered these groups it started to change how she felt about her body and her sexuality. She began to feel sexy and desired. For this group of women, involvement in alternative sexual lifestyles seemed to provide confidence and sexual empowerment.

Body Positive Activities

There are additional ways that these women were able to shift the reflection in the looking-glass, such as through activities like yoga, massage therapy, belly dancing, and exercise. The first excerpt from Claire indicates that she intentionally sought out yoga to help improve her self-image.

> I'm trying to do things to improve my self-image, like I've been doing a lot of yoga recently. And actually have started to see a yoga therapist. So trying to do like exercise that is not seen as a punishment, and you know, is helpful physically and mentally, and doesn't necessarily have the goal of like weight loss. Like just doing it for health benefits and well being—physical and mental. (Claire, 35, single)

It is clear from the quote above that Claire is still in the process of accepting her body, but she said that she is feeling better. It is incredibly difficult to overcome the years of fatphobic messages. Claire had a negative association with exercise because she saw it as connected to weight loss or punishment and the messages she received about needing to change her body to make it more acceptable and attractive. She hopes that by improving her self-image she will also improve her sexual agency and confidence.

Michelle is also in the process of improving her self-image through physical activity. When we spoke, Michelle had recently gone through a fairly trying divorce. Her husband was 'addicted to online pornography' and it destroyed their marriage. Michelle explained that even though she knew that his pornography addiction was not related to her appearance, she said she could not help but occasionally feel that if she were better looking or thinner that he would not have sought out sex online. When I asked her what she was doing that was making her feel better about herself, she told me that she was exercising regularly and had gone back to school to finish her bachelor's degree.

> I am relatively active, and I am far more active now than I ever was, probably. I swim several times a week, and I walk all over campus, and all of that kind of stuff. (Michelle, 27, divorced)

For Michelle the combination of going back to school and exercising has been instrumental in helping her overcome the numerous negative feelings she had about her body and self.

Katrina, 31 and single, also described finding an activity that not only has helped her improve her fitness level, but that has also helped her change the way she sees her body. Katrina joined a belly-dancing troupe, and eventually she and a friend started their own belly-dancing troupe. Katrina described the ways that the crowd responds to them, but her more specifically. She said that people line up after the performances to talk to her and that they typically tell her how beautiful she is. Katrina would like to lose weight, but performing as a belly dancer has helped her self-esteem tremendously. Similar to those in the kink community, belly dancing has provided a space where her body has ceased to be a social marker. Katrina is a large woman, and she said that she knows that she will never be "tiny." However, she said she is more realistic about her goals and she now appreciates what her body does for her and she feels more attractive than she did prior to learning to belly dance, which has made her more agentic in her sexual relationships.

Adoring Partners

Loving, adoring partners provide an excellent path toward feeling better about one's body. For some women it was their husband or partner who helped them find beauty in their bodies, but for others it was a less serious sexual relationship.

> But he loved every part of me. He would lay in the bed with me and he would squeeze the fat roll around my waist and I'll never forget it, the way it felt the first time he said, "I love your fat. I love this. I love how it feels against my skin." And that changed everything. It undid so much of the damage that had been done to me my whole life. Just those words, and knowing that as he looked at me he was completely serious and utterly sincere when he looked in my eyes and told me that. (Tracey, 32, divorced)

As is evident in Tracey's words, her lover changed the way she saw herself. She said that through his affection and sincerity she was able to overcome years of internalized fat hatred.

Becky, quoted below, also talked about a man who has helped change the way she sees herself. Becky noted that she has had difficulty in the past feeling comfortable sexually with men, especially at her current size (450 pounds).

> Yeah, so he was the first person who really took enough time to have me come, and played with all different parts of my body, and really I got a lot of belly acceptance, because my particular build is I carry most of my weight in front, in my belly. So you know, some people have more of an hourglass shape. I really don't, I have a comparably flat butt for my size, and he just really had a lot of different ways of expressing his tenderness and emotion and experimenting and playing around, it was just wonderful. (Becky, 32, divorced)

Her current partner is the first to spend the time she needed to reach orgasm and he has also helped her change the reflection she sees in the mirror because he pays attention to her body, especially her stomach, which she was especially self-conscious about.

Numerous women I interviewed for this project talked with me about the importance of a lover who paid attention to their bodies and made them feel beautiful, sexy, and wanted (see also Gailey, forthcoming). In the quote below, Mindy talks about two things that changed how she felt about her body: age and loving relationships. When Mindy and I spoke she was nine months pregnant and recently married. Mindy explained that as she has gotten older she has become more confident and assertive in her sexual relationships. She said that when she was young she was too concerned with how she looked and how the guy felt, now she's more concerned about enjoying the experience and less focused on how her body looks.

> As an adult I've become a lot more comfortable with my body and I think a lot of that has to do with just acceptance as an adult, but also having loving relationships with men who have told me that I'm beautiful, that they think that my body's fine. (Mindy, 40, married)

Elizabeth told me that before she was married she attended BBW and fat acceptance events with relative frequency because it was the perfect way to meet men who really liked to have sex with fat women. In the excerpt below she is telling me about her one of her best experiences with a man she met a size acceptance event.

> He loved big girls, everything about them, you name it. He loved full bush down in the vaginal area because big girls can't reach all of that so they don't worry about it. He loved all of that. He wanted a natural, all the little things that you would think, "Who could really find that attractive?" He loved it. Arm jiggle, rolls. He was into everything. I did not have to worry about one single physical thing with him, nothing. Even in sex. There's a lot of positions big girls can't do and the man ends up doing a lot of the work and all that kind of stuff and I used to feel bad about that. I would always force myself to do something physical while having sex. With him he liked doing all of that. It's all those little things. (Elizabeth, 30, married)

All those little things made a tremendous difference in Elizabeth's ability to enjoy sex and find pleasure in her own body. She told me that it used to make her nervous if she had sex with someone she thought had never had sex with a woman her size because he might be surprised by the fact that she did not shave or wax her pubic hair, that he would have to move folds of flesh to find her vulva, or that certain positions were not possible or were too difficult.

With Age Comes Body Acceptance

The women who were the youngest, under 25 or so, reported the most difficulty meeting partners, enjoying sex, and feeling confident undressing in the presence of a partner. Women in their late 30s and beyond were the most comfortable and some of them directly attributed the change in their comfort levels to their age (see also Gailey, forthcoming), as Mindy discussed above.

> When I was younger, I'm apple shaped, so my biggest part of me is my middle and when I was younger I would so not connect with my body. I would just see

> my head. If I touched my belly I'd snatch my hand back like I'd scalded it. I just pretended it wasn't there. Now I'm in this process of really being in my belly if that makes any sense. (Brooke, 35, married)

Brooke's account of the difference between how she felt when she was young and how she feels now was a common experience for many of the women. Like so many of the women I talked with, Brooke used to live "from the neck up," meaning that she only paid attention to her face and tried to dissociate from her body. Brooke is becoming increasingly comfortable disrobing in front of her husband now that she is consciously trying to "be in her belly" or embody her fat.

Cathy, like so many other women I interviewed, also indicated that her view of her body and own attractiveness is better and so are her sexual experiences.

> I think I'm attractive and now there is someone else who thinks I'm attractive. It was more of a positive and more positive as far as the physical experience too. I mean when I was doing that when I was in college most of my sexual experiences were not very positive. (Cathy, 44, divorced)

Cathy explained that her experiences in college were not positive because she was insecure about her body and was not sure how the men would react to her.

A common sentiment among these women was that they felt that as fat women they had to put aside their own sexual satisfaction and needs because they feared that if they did not focus solely on the men that they were having intercourse with that the men would no longer be interested in them. As they got older, they realized that this mindset was flawed and that they also needed to respect their own needs during a sexual encounter (Gailey, forthcoming).

Women who accept their bodies, or are beginning to, not only experience freedom from the pressure to diet or change their bodies, but also the freedom to be sexual. As the women experience less body shame and increased confidence, they also seek out or attract partners who treat them better and truly appreciate them (Gailey, 2012). Participants who have begun to see their bodies as beautiful and desired seem to enjoy their sexual relationships and have better experiences than those who do not.

Discussion and Conclusion

The present study indicates that it is possible for numerous large women, not just those associated with the size acceptance community (Gailey, 2012), to overcome at least some the self-hatred associated with fat. It was apparent from the interviews that there are multiple life experiences that have helped set the stage for learning to appreciate and accept one's body—that is, transforming the looking-glass. For many, online dating opened up a door that had previously been closed because it showed these women that there are partners who are attracted to fat women who are not fat fetishists or men who think that fat women are "easy" (Prohaska and Gailey, 2009). This was described as an important turning point because they felt it was nearly impossible to meet potential partners the way their "thin" friends do. But, it was not just online dating that led to sexual empowerment. Involvement in the kink community, engagement in body positive activities, adoring partners, and the process of aging all helped lead these women down a path toward bodily acceptance and sexual empowerment.

Body image is tremendously important for women's enjoyment in sexual relationships (Hoyt and Kogan, 2002), and previous research has shown that "when women accept their bodies they tend to become more agentic in their sexuality" (Gailey, 2012, p. 115). Unfortunately, research is limited with respect to body image and sexual satisfaction among mid-life women. A couple of studies have shown that as women age they experience greater sexual satisfaction and less body anxiety (Tiggerman and Lynch, 2002; Stephenson and Meston, 2012), but others point to the increasing dissatisfaction women feel with their bodies as they 'age out' of attractiveness (Clarke and Griffin, 2008).

There is so much pressure on women in Western cultures to meet the excruciatingly narrow beauty standards that it is practically heresy for a woman to be happy with her body—especially a fat woman. Women are taught to hate their bodies and that there is always something they can change to improve their appearance (Wolf, 2002). The dominant discourse suggests that people have control over their body shape and size through either hard work or through the consumption of goods and services. It is really easy to be influenced by the dominant ideology that women should strive to look "perfect" or embody "emphasized femininity," and most women report some degree of dissatisfaction with their bodies (Bordo, 2004; Hesse-Biber, 2007).

The women that I spoke with, for the most part, did not believe that they fit the conventional beauty mandate and felt subversive when they were pleased with their appearance. This is likely because fat is perceived as a threat to the heteronormative system because it challenges the gender order and transgresses norms for both men and women's behaviors in sexual relationships. Unfortunately, this research is limited to heterosexual encounters. Future research should focus on same-sex relationships to further understand the role partners play in the embodiment of fat acceptance.

Embodiment of fat helps women subvert the larger societal view that fat women are either nonsexual or hypersexual (Gailey, 2014). It was not necessary for women to subscribe to size acceptance as Gailey's (2012) research showed as long as they found other ways that they could change the reflection in the looking-glass. Frequently it was not through weight loss or any other physical change—it was the way they think about and see their body and their self-worth that needed to change. Embodiment of fat involved a process whereby these women have found ways to make their bodies sexual on their own terms.

References

Bacon, L., 2010. *Health at every size: The surprising truth about your weight.* 2nd edition. BenBella Books.

Blank, H., 2000. *Big big love: A sourcebook on sex for people of size and those who love them.* CA: Greenery Press.

Boero, N., 2012. *Killer fat: Media, medicine, and morals in the American "obesity epidemic."* New Jersey: Rutgers University Press.

Bordo, S., 2004. *Unbearable Weight: Feminism, Western Culture, and the Body.* California: University of California Press.

Charmaz, K., and Mitchell R., 2001. Grounded theory in ethnography. In: Atkinson, A. Coffey, S. Delamont, J. Lofland, and L. Lofland, eds. 2001. *Handbook of ethnography*, London: Sage Publications, pp. 160–176.

Clarke, L. H. and Griffin, M., 2008. Visible and invisible ageing: Beauty work as a response to ageism. *Aging & Society*, 28, 653–674.

Connell, R.W., 1987. *Gender and power.* Stanford, CA: Stanford University Press.

Cooley, C. H., 1902. *Human nature and the social order.* New York: Scribner's.

Ernsberger, P., 2009. Does social class explain the connection between weight and health? In: E. Rothblum and S. Solovay, eds. *The fat studies reader*, New York: New York University Press, pp. 25–36.

Finkel, E. J., Eastwick, P. W., Karney, B. R., Reis, H. T., and S. Sprecher, S., 2012. Online dating: A critical analysis from the perspective of psychological science. *Psychological Science in the Public Interest*, pp. 1–64.

Gailey, J. A., 2014. *The hyper(in)visible fat woman: Weight and gender discourse in contemporary society.* New York: Palgrave Macmillan.

Gailey, J. A., 2012. Fat shame to fat pride: Fat women's sexual and dating experiences. *Fat Studies*, 1(1), pp. 114–127.

Gailey, J. A. and Prohaska, A., 2006. 'Knocking off a fat girl': An exploration of hogging, male sexuality, and neutralizations. *Deviant Behavior*, 27, pp. 31–49.

Glaser, B. G. and Strauss, A. C., 1967. *The discovery of grounded theory: Strategies for qualitative research.* Aldine Transaction.

Goffman, E., 1963. *Stigma: Notes on the management of a spoiled identity.* New Jersey: Prentice-Hall.

Goode, E. and Preissler, J., 1983. The fat admirer. *Deviant Behavior*, 4, pp. 175–202.

Harris, M. B., 1990. Is love seen as different for the obese? *Journal of Applied Social Psychology*, 20, pp. 1209–1224.

Hesse-Biber, S. N., 2007. *The cult of thinness.* New York: Oxford University Press.

Hoyt, W. D. and Kogan, L. R. 2002. Satisfaction with body image and peer relationships for males and females in a college environment. *Sex Roles*, 45, pp. 199–215.

Lupton, D., 2012. *Fat.* London: Routledge.

Murray, S., 2004. Locating aesthetics: Sexing the fat woman. *Social Semiotics*, 14, pp. 237–247.

Newmahr, S., 2011. *Playing on the edge: Sadomasochism, risk, and intimacy.* Bloomington: Indiana University Press.

Patrick, H., Neighbors, C., and Knee, C. R., 2004. Appearance-related social comparisons: The role of contingent self-esteem and self-perceptions of attractiveness. *Personality and Social Psychology Bulletin*, 30, pp. 501–514.

Prohaska, A. and Gailey, J. A., 2009. Fat women as 'easy targets': Achieving masculinity through hogging. In: E. Rothblum and S. Solovay, eds. *The fat studies reader*, New York: New York University Press, pp. 158–166.

Regan, P. C., 1996. Sexual outcasts: The perceived impact of body weight and gender on sexuality. *Journal of Applied Social Psychology*, 26, pp. 1803–1815.

Satinsky, S., Dennis, B., Reece, M. Sanders, S., and Bardzell, S., 2013. My 'fat girl complex': A preliminary invesitgation of sexual health and body image in women of size. *Culture, Health & Sexuality: An International Journal for Research, Intervention and Care,* DOI: 10.1080/13691058.2013.783236.

Stephenson, K. R. and Meston, C. M., 2012. The young and the restless: Age as a moderator of the association between sexual desire and sexual distress in women. *Journal of Sex & Marital Therapy*, 38, pp. 445–457.

Swami, V. and Tovèe, M. J., 2009. Big beautiful women: The body size preferences of male fat admirers. *Journal of Sex Research*, 46, pp. 89–96.

Tiggerman, M. and Lynch, J. E., 2002. Body image across the life span in adult women: The role of objectification. *Developmental Psychology*, 37, pp. 243–253.

Turner, B. S. 1996. *The Body and Society.* 2nd ed. Sage Publications, Inc.

Waskul, D. D. and Vannini, P., 2006. Introduction: The body in symbolic interaction. In: D. Waskul and P. Vannini ed. *Body/embodiment: Symbolic interaction and the sociology of the body.* Aldershot: Ashgate, pp. 1–18.

Weinstein, R. J., 2012. *Fat sex: The naked truth.* Self published.

Wolf, N., 2002. *The beauty myth: How images of beauty are used against women.* Harper Perennial, Reprint Edition.

Chapter 5

Against "Good Taste": Class, Corpulence and the Subversive Pleasures of "Unfit" Femininities

Frances Hatherley

Introduction

The forms of oppression against women are multiple and interconnected, my intention for this chapter is to contribute new knowledge to the field of fat studies by exploring the intersections of fat and class. Much in the vein of feminist fat activists' project of reclaiming the word fat, as Marilyn Wann states "as a preferred political identity" (2009, p. xii), the wish here is that by appropriating some of the negative descriptions launched at the working-class fat body, their power to shame will be subverted.

The word *corpulence* speaks of more than just fat; it describes a body that is an overabundance, of almost pure corporeality. Its very bodiliness strongly connects it to the lower stratum, of the vulgar and the base. Likewise, the working-class body shares many of these cultural associations with lowness and dirt. Therefore this chapter attempts to make room for another word alongside fat for describing flesh, with its added political weight of connotations behind it. The use of the word corpulent encourages a willful *lowering* of ourselves to play with the pleasures of vulgarity, to revel in the bodily, to hopefully begin to look at the body and class distinctions in a new light away from bourgeois value judgements surrounding working-class female bodies and fat bodies alike.

In 1978, Susie Orbach wrote that "fat is a feminist issue." Today in the British media it is also a strongly-marked issue of class. On television, in papers and films, in everyday conversation, the working-class body has become a site of disgust, with millionaires like Jamie Oliver and right-wing politicians using society's fear of the fleshy, corpulent body as a moralizing stick to beat the poor. Fatness is used as visual shorthand to signify the working-classes' supposed bad spending, bad eating habits, and—in short—"bad taste." The image of the working-class in the British popular imagination has morphed from one of hard-working respectability to a *body* that is hated, despised and ridiculed: a body on which is written a brash, distasteful, lazy ignorance, a body seen as physically and socially "unfit." Nowhere is this more true than in the case of the fat *female* working-class body. Fat women's visible rejection of the discipline of bodily regulation is taken as evidence of a scandalous irresponsibility, a loss of control over the self and its physical boundaries.

The "overweight," "out of control" body has been lampooned with shocking brutality by shows such as *Little Britain* (UK, 2003–2006), and poked and prodded at in health-food, exercise and lifestyle programs as an illustration of how *not* to be/eat/dress/look. Everywhere, "excessive" flesh is taken as a sign of moral deficiency—and the image of fleshy excess is most often *female*. Tellingly, in Owen Jones's *Chavs* (2011) the case studies discussed are predominately ample-bodied women, such as the fictional character Vicky Pollard and the real-life Shannon Mathews and Jade Goody; and yet Jones's analysis, although sympathetic towards gendered issues, makes no attempt to analyse *why* the demonization of working-class women so often targets their bodies, far more so than for men.

I am interested in what it is about the fat female body that provokes such hatred. Fat and poverty are now firmly coupled in the imagination of today's media culture in the UK. By depicting the working-class body as stereotypically fat, we frame it as out of bounds, out of control, undisciplined: fat here is the personification of the unruly masses of the "lumpen" proletariat. However, our cultural fear of fat runs deeper than a distaste for junk food and infirm bodies: it says something particularly about the way we view women. For fat in these discourses is also a signifier of female abundance gone unchecked. In *Letting Ourselves Go* (2001) Celia Hartley explores the connections of sexism and sizeism:

> Women who do not maintain rigid control over the boundaries of their bodies, allowing them to become large and "unfeminine," are treated with derision in our society, and that derision is tied inextricably to the personal freedom of women. Women who are fat are said to have "let themselves go." The very phrase connotes a losing of restraints. Women in our society are bound. (Hartley, 2001, p. 63)

What Hartley suggests then is that the fat female body performs femininity incorrectly and is in breach of the social contract that enforces a normative gender appearance. The socially stigmatized "unfit" female body appears at the intersection of class and gender, framed by media and visual culture as an unruly object requiring constant self-surveillance, maintenance and work.

In this chapter I turn to Michel Foucault's theories on biopolitics and social discipline, and Pierre Bourdieu's work in "distinction" and "good taste," to explore how social judgements around taste and the body take on a political meaning. I also discuss the sociological research of Beverly Skeggs into the ways working-class women have historically been encouraged to adopt middle-class forms of "respectability" in a performance of class-passing. However, my intention is not only to challenge negative representations of a female working-class corpulence, but also to explore the ways in which the fat body, so often described as unattractive, and even as disgusting, can produce feelings of delight, familiarity and pleasure. To this end, I explore the links between the epicurean delights of food, feasting and sex, and the historical classing of the pleasures of the carnival.

I will proceed by exploring the themes of bodily discipline and normalized femininity, the connections between fat-shaming and chav-hate, and the connection of epicurean pleasures to sex and disgust. Disrupting the distinction between "high" and "low" culture, I draw on images from the spheres of fine art and pop culture in order to encourage a theoretical and imaginative seepage. Representing "low culture" are *The Fat Slags* from the comic *Viz*. These characters (or caricatures) have seldom been critically discussed, and when they are it is usually in terms of gender *or* class, without connecting the two in order to see how classist and sexist mockery converge on the fat female working-class body. From the world of fine art painting, I will be considering Jenny Saville's giant fat nudes. I'm particularly interested in images that take the notion of corpulent femininity as disgusting and subvert it, instead showing the ways in which we can take pleasure in what is culturally disavowed—in the fleshiness, supposed messiness and abjection of bodies that are against "good taste."

The Female Social Body: Disciplines of Discreetness and Respectability

In order to say *what it is* that is "against good taste," it is worth outlining some of the ways the body and its performance of femininity have been constructed in terms of discourses on *distinction*. Those women who have managed to *pull off* the appearance of possessing "good taste" have somehow got *being a woman* correct—a performance often described as being/looking "feminine," "classy," "lady-like," "sophisticated" and so on. Although the trends of what is considered beautiful or stylish repeatedly shift, certain bodies have been largely excluded from mainstream celebration, appreciation and aspiration within the standards set within Western culture. The fleshy female body has remained a site of crisis and conflict. As Susie Orbach says of our preoccupation with body image, "In the discourse about self-created identity, the body is central. It is central because it is a vehicle to assert one's place as a member of a class, a group, a sexual practice, an aspiration. It is central because it is a place of anxiety itself" (2009, p. 142). As I will go on to argue, it is often a result of these social anxieties that the powerful erotics of fat sex are disavowed.

The effects of social and political power, which sets standards to live up to, shape the ways in which we view and inhabit our bodily realities. One of the main points of Michel Foucault's discussion of biopolitics in *Discipline and Punish* (1991) is that bodies are not simply a result of nature and biology alone, but a product of the enforcement of power, socially constructed under a discipline imposed by the state apparatus. Foucault's notion of the "docile body" here helps us to imagine how notions of what it means to have good taste, to be feminine, beautiful or classy, hold such sway with us, to the point that our bodies are actively shaped by such distinctions. The "docile body" is the body made historically malleable by cultural fashioning—in Foucault's words, by "a policy of coercions that act upon the body, a calculated manipulation of its elements, its gestures, its behaviours … a machinery of power that explores [the body], breaks it down and rearranges it" (Foucault, 1991, pp. 135–169). But power according to Foucault also generates its own resistance: the docile body is not simply tamed, but involved in ongoing conflicts against the desire to control and normalize it.

The theory that our bodily tastes and behaviours are *learned* and socialized constructs is the subject of the sociologist and philosopher Pierre Bourdieu's 1979 book *Distinction: A Social Critique of the Judgement of Taste.* Bourdieu's work can be used to illuminate an argument that is often taken for granted: that judgements that "distinguish" those that possess "good taste" discriminate against those that do not. Bourdieu argues that "taste, a class culture turned into nature, that is, *embodied*, helps to shape the class body." (Bourdieu, 2010, p. 188)—ideas of good taste proliferate down from ideology to shape the very bodies of socially classed subjects. A key aspect of Bourdieu's thesis is that those possessing "distinction" are equipped with a form of knowledge that privileges them: their knowledge is a form of cultural-capital that helps to advance their social and financial position in life as well as the workplace. As a privilege of the upper and middle-classes, "taste" is passed on to their children as well as being repeated in their schooling. This contradicts the common notion that it is being "naturally smart" that enables people to get on in life. As Owen Jones argues:

> Being born into a prosperous middle-class family typically endows you with a safety net for life. If you are not naturally very bright, you are still likely to go far and, at the very least, will never experience poverty as an adult. A good education compounded by your parents' "cultural capital," financial support and networks will always see you through. If you are a bright child born into a working-class family, you do not have any of these things. The odds are that you will not be better off than your parents. Britain's class system is like an invisible prison. (Jones, 2011, p. 182)

Although there isn't the space here to discuss educational inequality *per se*, it is worth mentioning the role of privileged education in endowing people with class-based cultural-capital, a seemingly effortless awareness of "good taste." My argument here is not that "working-class taste" is better than "bourgeois taste," but that the latter sets the rules and the former follows them: for many working-class women, failing to live up to the standards of taste risks social stigma, the loss of status and with it respectability.

The idea that there was once a positive identity available to the working-class, a notion of the "respectable working-class," has largely disappeared from British cultural memory. In its place is a blame-the-victim strategy which systematically discredits the existence of soaring social inequality through negative representations of the working-class as lazy, criminal, disobedient, uneducated, slobs—in other words, as "chavs." Yet respectability still matters to working-class women, as Bev Skeggs shows in *Formations of Class and Gender: Becoming Respectable.* Skeggs uses decades of field work and interviews with working-class women in the UK to show how important is it for people to feel that despite being poor they are hard-working and decent—and, more poignantly, that they are *respectable.*

Skeggs's findings suggest that many women equate respectability with being middle/upper-class. Considering working-class women's motivations for cultivating respectability, Skeggs argues that "respectability is one of the most ubiquitous signifiers of class" and "one of the key mechanisms by which some groups were 'othered' and pathologised" (Skeggs, 1997, p. 1). While "rarely recognised as an issue by those who are positioned within it," respectability is "usually the concern of those who are seen not to have it": the "working-classes (Black and White)" who have "consistently been classified as dangerous, polluting, threatening, revolutionary, pathological and without respect" (Skeggs, 1997, p. 1). This is not to say that middle-class women do not feel social pressure, but that due to their class positions a level of respectability is already assumed. Whereas, working-class women and women of colour have the types of discrimination Skeggs mentions to push against, always having to prove something rather than it be taken for granted.

For women of all classes, the body is a form of cultural capital: having a correctly "docile body," a body that is shaped in adherence to the beauty norms of Western culture, can make the difference between inclusion and exclusion. Much hangs on the successful performance of feminine good taste, seen both morally and aesthetically, i.e. the fear of being described as dressing "trashy" is a fear of being thought of as being literally worthless rubbish. As Skeggs points out, working-class women have been identified with *pollution*: the poor are seen as "the masses," a rabble which is politically dangerous to the ruling-class *status quo*. This pollution and danger is also connected to dangerous sexuality, so that poverty is yoked to lowness and baseness, seen as both physically and metaphysically "dirty."

A historical sketch of the way femininity became connected with class position is given by Skeggs:

> the emergence of femininity as an ideal was produced through textuality in the eighteenth century. The femininity produced had an affinity with the habitus of the upper-classes, of ease, restraint, calm and luxurious decoration. It was produced as a sign of difference from other women [. . .] Femininity was seen to be the *property* of the middle-class women who could *prove* themselves to be respectable through their appearance. Because femininity developed as a classed sign it became imbued with different amounts of power. (1997, p. 99)

This highlights the power struggles for women to get femininity right, as to get it wrong as Skeggs points out is a blow to the already weakened position of women in society, pitting women against each other in the struggle for social standing.

For working-class women, access to femininity and good taste calls for a form of class-passing in order to *pull off* the behaviors, dress and tastes of those with power: the habitus of the middle and upper classes must be aped, or at best appropriated. Speaking of the attitudes of the young women she interviewed, Skeggs notes, "Class was central to the young women's subjectivities. It was not spoken of in the traditional sense of recognition—I am working-class—but rather, was displayed in their multitudinous efforts *not to be* recognized as working-class. They disidentified and they dissimulated." (original italics, Skeggs, 1997, p. 74). Therefore, in seeking social validation and visibility, many women felt they needed to disavow their class background.

The idea of "good taste," of who has it and who doesn't, has always been used by politicians, media personalities and comedians to mock and degrade the existence of the working-classes. This "chav-hate" has reached fever pitch of late—just think of Jamie Oliver referring with anger and revulsion to poor British families eating "chips and cheese out of Styrofoam containers" while sitting in a room with a "massive fucking TV" (Deans, 2013). Here are the ultimate signifiers of bad taste: the *unacceptable* incongruous mixing of very cheap food with very expensive luxury goods. Why should these families have what he himself undoubtedly enjoys, when they didn't *earn* it? There is a strong element of hypocritical moral shaming going on here, a concern about people living within their means, which a millionaire like Jamie Oliver perhaps doesn't have to worry about. But what I think is really going on here, what the revulsion expresses, is an extreme distaste towards the pleasures sought by the working-classes. As Owen Jones says of the word "chav":

> Many use it to show their distaste towards working-class people who have embraced consumerism, only to spend their money in supposedly tacky and uncivilised ways rather than the discreet elegance of the bourgeoisie. (Jones, 2011, p. 8)

This is not fundamentally about healthy eating, or the supposed obesity epidemic (let's also bear in mind the indulgences also shared by the middle-classes, be they drugs, drinking or dangerous crash/fad dieting, which hardly set a healthy example), but about policing those pleasures that do not conform to bourgeois standards of refinement and food as expressions of cultural capital.

Good taste can thus be seen to function as a tool of social normalization, a way in which we are encouraged to conform by performing the only *proper* way of being feminine, respectable and worthy of status. It is time here to examine the influence of media images of women on women's self-image, and their inscription of oppressive beauty norms onto the bodies and psyches of women as if they were "in the market" themselves. What I want to draw out here is the ways in which the corpulent body breaches the social boundaries of "good taste," refusing the social disciplines of state power: this body stands in the way of control.

Defining Femininity and the Normalization of the Body out of Bounds

I will now turn to an exploration of the function of *aspirational femininity* as a clever tool for social discipline, in that it appears to come from one's internal desire rather than external pressures, promoting self-regulation as a lifestyle choice. The images of women in western culture's media are more often than not depicting an aspiration which links the body with the capitalist economy of attainment and improvement, shaping women's attitudes to their own bodily realities from the inside out.

The influence of photography's claim to realism, used to advertise diet food, cosmetics and clothing in the 1980s and 90s is interrogated by Susan Bordo in *Unbearable Weight: Feminism, Western Culture and The Body* (1993). On these images Bordo remarks, "the ideal here is of a body that is absolutely tight, contained, 'bolted down,' firm: in other words, a body that is protected against eruption from within, whose internal processes are under control. Areas that are soft, loose, or 'wiggly' are unacceptable, even on extremely thin bodies." (1993, pp. 190–91). The products advertised promise to reign in *out of control* flesh, and in doing so posit our own natural bodily states as horrific, as something to regulate and fight against. Anybody that isn't firm or slender is *excessive* and *bad*: flesh itself comes to be viewed as if it were abjection or waste (the concept of abjection theorized by Julia Kristeva (1984) will be taken up later in this chapter to account for the fears and fascination attached to fat sexuality).

Seen in the mirror of aspirational femininity, the female body is a site of constant anxiety: never enough, never complete, but a perpetual site of improvement and regulation. The young and slender body type is held up as the epitome of acceptable femaleness, not only praised as beautiful but used as a symbol of success. This ideal body type is used to market products, clothes, cosmetics and lifestyles, with the promise that they will get us nearer to the goal of *successful* femininity—which, it is implied, will guarantee happiness and fulfilment. It is represented as class-neutral, but unattainable to anybody who cannot afford the products that will help one on the way to perfection.

Bordo's research is supported by Susie Orbach's work as an analyst with women with serious body dysphoria. In *Bodies* (2009), Orbach illustrates the ways women are, in a real sense, bullied into conforming to the ideal feminine type. Women are made to fear that one wrong move out of the realm of bodily desirability will lead to the loss of their identity, in a society in which only correct body types are given visibility and representation. Orbach outlines how the fear of being marginalized or getting *being a woman* wrong becomes the learnt behavior of anxious self-surveillance, which women inadvertently pass on in their judgments of other women:

> [A] woman's body, we learn, is not a very good or safe environment to live inside. Rarely are our mothers and other female adults able to convey to a young woman that her body, whatever natural shape it has, is a source of pride and of beauty, since they themselves have not been able to feel that. We learn instead that our bodies are powerful in a negative sense, they destabilise men and get us into trouble. It is no wonder that we become frightened of our bodies and see them not as where we live but as part of us that we must control, watch and direct. (Orbach, 2009, p. 164)

According to Bordo and Orbach, the levels of eating disorders, body dysphoria and cosmetic surgery in Western societies have never been higher. We seem to be increasingly frightened of bodily realities that transgress boundaries. These boundaries can be physical, as in the case of a body that is large, takes up space and cannot be confined to "regular" clothing sizes. They can also be *metaphysical*, to do with rules of "good taste" and ideals of feminine discreetness. The corpulent body, whose markers of difference are highly visible and represent to patriarchy a body that has become frighteningly formless, breaches both kinds of boundary. Bordo underlines the enormity of this terror:

> when 500 people were asked what they feared most in the world, 190 replied, 'getting fat.' In an age when our children regularly have nightmares of nuclear

> holocaust, that as adults we should give *this* answer—that we most fear 'getting fat'—is far more bizarre than the anorexic's misperceptions of her body image, or the bulimic's compulsive vomiting. (Bordo, 1993, p. 141)

Yet in many ways this is not "bizarre" at all, it is the logical and very real threat of ostracism in a society that manipulates women by provoking terror of their own bodies: fear of fat is really a fear of stigmatization.

The treatment of the corpulent body mirrors that of class: both are repeatedly erased from visual culture, disavowed and suppressed in favour of a kind of universalized slim, discreet, class-neutral subject. Now that being fat and being working-class are irrevocably tied together in the popular imagination, fatness is a visible stain, a class stigma. Because being working-class no longer carries any positive identification, as Skeggs notes, working-class women want to *disidentify* with it, to escape becoming an object of ridicule and hate (Skeggs, 1997). The pleasingly-plump body that speaks of health and vigour has been disavowed, and is seen instead as a body that has failed to keep itself in correct (social) shape. It reveals unhealthy appetites, a lack of moral and physical discipline, as Skeggs argues:

> The working-class body which is signalled through fat is one that has given up the hope of ever 'improving,' of becoming middle-class. It is the body which is recognised for what it is: a working-class body that is beyond the regulation and disciplines required to be part of social and cultural exchanges. (1997, p. 82)

Therefore, these intersections of oppressions mean that the poor and fleshy are demonized as doubly failing.

Failing to "improve," to pass as middle-class, means being denied access to social power but also, and perhaps more insidiously, being shut out from femininity itself. As Carol-Anne Tyler says in *Female Impersonation:* "A real woman is a real lady, otherwise she is a female impersonator, whose 'unnaturally bad' taste—like that attributed to working-class women or women of colour —marks the impersonation as such" (Tyler, 2002, p. 61). To quote "Susan," a woman interviewed by Beverly Skeggs: "To them *you never fit*, never up to their standards" (Skeggs, 1997 p. 3, my italics). It is important for us then to reject these standards and take pleasure in that which is deemed "unfit," to subvert bourgeois tastes and value judgments that decide who is "good" enough.

I am not interested here in learning how we might better pass, but in how we might *enjoy* that which we have been taught to abhor. By understanding the threat the corpulent body poses to the standards of attractive and correct femaleness promoted through visual culture and the media, we learn how powerful the presence of that body is in its double rebelliousness. In the next section I explore some stereotypical representations of the corpulent body's supposedly insatiable appetites, and its connotations of working-class deviancy and promiscuity. Although such deviancy is most commonly presented through a bourgeois moralistic framing, here I will attempt to reclaim a carnivalesque figure that for many of us is a source of rebellious delight, as well as sensual pleasure.

Against Fat Shaming and Chav-Hate: Enjoying *The Fat Slags*

Created by Graham Dury, *The Fat Slags* first came to life in 1989 in a comic strip in the British (adult) comic *Viz*. Although The *Fat Slags* seem to conform to all of the negative stereotypes associated with working-class female sexuality, I want to argue for a subversive rereading of them. The strip depicts its eponymous heroines, Sandra Burke and Tracey Tunstall (or San and Tray), in their debaucherous and carnivalesque adventures with their lover Baz and his bin-man mate Dave. The pair, sometimes with Baz or Dave in tow, romp about satisfying their prodigious appetites and pursuing lecherous schemes. A strong theme of the comedy, the core joke of their (mis)adventures, is of class passing: they pursue what they *think* are the signifiers of respectable femininity and desirability.

It is worth contrasting Sandra and Tracey with *Little Britain*'s (2003–2006) Vicky Pollard. Like Sandra and Tracey, Vicky Pollard is *unfit,* both fat and highly sexed: one persistent joke is how many kids she has by how many fathers. The audience's laughter at her feckless, stupid and aggressive behavior is vitriolic and derisive: we are positioned not only as knowing more than her, but as intrinsically superior: when she "gets it wrong," it is because she is simply "thick." But much of the humor of *The Fat Slags* derives from our *enjoyment* of their brazen shamelessness in trying to get away with it, while another part comes from the way their mishaps draw attention to the often ridiculous nature of distinction itself, the arbitrariness of the lines that separate good taste from bad. When Tracy and Sandra "get it wrong," it is often because what is being aimed at is itself unachievable for most women, whatever class they are.

This is why I find *The Fat Slags* so subversive: there is no attempt to toe the line and conform to bourgeois norms of bodily discipline and sexual discretion—these are totally cast off. This is not to say that Tracy and Sandra are wholly radical figures: there is also nastiness, stupidity and grotesque humiliation. In the story *The Pudding Club* (Dury and Thorp, 1994), Tracey thinks Sandra might be pregnant, so they go to the chemist to purchase a pregnancy test. Sandra says to Tracey "Eh? Fucking 'hell. Are you up the duff Tray?" to which Tracey replies "No y'gormless cunt … you are … at least I think you are … Ere! G'behind the shampoo rack and piss on this stick" (p. 6). In the next scene we see Sandra's huge, perfectly round bottom sticking out the end of the aisle, and a large pool of piss spreading across the floor. This scene is rich with the low pleasures of totally shameless lewdness. Certain protocols of social discreetness *are* being attempted—Sandra does try to go discreetly behind the aisle—but her large bottom pokes out, and everyone can see she is "doing it" where she's not meant to be "doing it."

There is humiliation and abjection here, but at the same time Sandra's failure to "get it right" flies in the face of our moralization about bodily functions that must be kept private. However, we are never allowed to fully sympathize with the *Slags*. For example, Sandra decides that now she's pregnant she'd "best start smoking low tar" (Dury and Thorp, 1994, pp. 6–14) and will switch from rum and coke to rum and orange juice; when told she won't be able to go to the pub after having the baby, she immediately decides to give it up for adoption. Obviously this is problematic: the flagging up and exaggerating of these stereotypes to grotesque degrees expresses an ambivalent stance on who is being made a fool of. And yet, in our current climate of chav-hating and fat shaming, representations of abundantly fleshy libidinous femininities, of women who enjoy eating as much as fucking and refuse to be shamed into invisibility, are most welcome. They force us to explore our society's class and gender discriminations, if not always standing as figures of rebellious resistance.[1]

Tracy and Sandra's vigorous sexuality plays with stereotypes that link the fat body with all things *bodily:* its processes and desires are those of a body that seeps, expands, devours and absorbs, a body whose appetites are various and voracious. As mentioned earlier, the fleshy body that doesn't display the strict boundaries of slim discreetness is often treated as if monstrous. The social fear of becoming fat, of losing social status and visibility becomes sublimated into a terror of appetite itself (see Pat Lyons's 2009 text *Prescription for Harm* for a further discussion of the negative effects and failures of the diet industry). But these suppressed bodily appetites burst out as the polymorphous desires of the carnival—desires for food and sex and the frowned-upon pleasures of drinking, smoking and profanity (the front cover of the 1994 *The Big Fat Slags Book* promises an "orgy of sex, chips and swearing"). The carnivalesque, as theorized by Mikhail Bakhtin in *Rabelais and His World* (1984), is a space where normal social conduct is temporarily abandoned in favour of the pleasures of food, drink and sex, of revelling in the low and base. Bakhtin also discusses a carnivalesque or "grotesque" body typified as feminine, a body that transgresses clear boundaries of inside and out, an actively functioning, sexual and visceral body. *The Fat Slags* are the epitome of this, which is the major source of their (and our) delight.

---

1 To see the cover of Viz's *The Big Fat Slags* book please visit: http://www.amazon.co.uk/The-Big-Fat-Slags-Book/dp/1870870468.

One facet of the sexual escapades of Tracey and Sandra is that they are not depicted as sexually naive or subservient to men's desire. Although not advocating that women pick men up and discard them whenever the mood takes them, as was promoted by the "Ladette" culture of the 1990s, I do find in *The Fat Slags* a subversive recasting of the gendered and classed sexual norms that cast the working-class male as a virile, highly sexed, swaggering partner. Fat sexuality is so often described in visual culture as something terrible and devouring, gobbling up unsuspecting males, for example, Hattie Jacques pursuing unwilling males in the British *Carry On* films from the 1970s. In mainstream media and visual culture it is represented as unwelcome—think of the supposedly comic sight of a fat woman being attracted to a male and going after the "poor bloke" like a shark with the scent of blood, while the male victim attempts to escape, perhaps towards a nice middle-class thin girl dressed demurely. In *The Fat Slags* this is not the case: in fact, Baz and Dave are extremely willing, desirous and somewhat easily-led partners.

What depictions of carnivalesque femininities such as those found in *The Fat Slags* so powerfully—and I must add deliciously—subvert is the push to reject the body in favour of the mind, to separate ourselves from the lowness of our own messiness and our inescapable mortality. To train our bodies out of the free pleasures of inhabiting them, our corporeal selves must be disavowed by the market-led disciplines that promote "being in shape," against the terrors of being considered "unfit." Rather than being shamed by our class or our bodies, we can see the corpulent female body as a site not of lack but of abundance, embodying some of our basic needs and pleasures. Before moving deeper into discussions of food, eating and their linkages to sex and sensuality, I'd like to end this section with a passage by Leslie Fielder:

> All of us have memories of having once been cuddled against the buxom breast and folded into the ample arms of a warm soft Giantess, whose bulk—to our 8-pound, 21-inch infant selves—must have seemed as mountainous as any 600-pound Fat Lady to our adult selves. And to rediscover in our latter loves the superabundance of female flesh which we remember from our first is surely a satisfaction we all project in dreams, though we may be unwilling to confess it once we are awake. (Fielder, 1978, p. 131)

The socially disallowed desire for fecund fleshiness, so often denied to our disciplined adult selves is with the help of projects like *Fat Sex: New Directions in Theory and Activism* (2015) coming back to prominence, to bring this desire out of the closet of our dreams.

Epicurean Pleasures and Appetites of Disgust: Linkages of Food and Sex

If our tastes are subject to social shaping then our pleasures are put under possibly even greater regulation. Here I will develop in more detail the discussion of classed eating habits which I started earlier with reference to the taste-policing of Jamie Oliver, focusing on the pleasures of eating, its relation to sex and sensuality and its classed dimensions. Finally, I will use the paintings of Jenny Saville to explore the powers and pleasures of viscerality and disgust.

It is a cruel irony that food being one of the most easily-accessible pleasures as well as vital sustenance, is symbolically held out at a distance from people. In *Cruel Optimism* Lauren Berlant comments, "Food is one of the few spaces of controllable, reliable pleasures people have. Additionally, unlike alcohol or other drugs, food is necessary to existence, part of the care of the self, the reproduction of life. But how do we articulate those urgencies of necessity and pleasure with the structural conditions of existence that militate against the flourishing of workers and consumers?" (2011, p. 115). What this has to do with class is that many middle-class "foodies" have treated the enjoyment of cheap food, often stodgy yet flavorsome and filling, as a low pleasure and a shameful indicator of bad taste. Berlant continues: "In short, every day more and more advice circulates from more locations about how better to get the fat (the substance and the people) under control" (2011, p. 103). Think of the aforementioned Jamie Oliver tirade as an example of this hypocritical policing of the lower class by the upper classes.

In many areas of the UK now without local market stalls selling fresh fruit, vegetables and fish cheaply, it is harder to access healthy, low fat foods on a budget. Cheap food from supermarkets is often heavily processed, containing lots of added fats, sugar and salt to bulk it up, making it cheaper to produce. On such diets it is not surprising that many poor people are getting fatter. It is true that it is possible to eat cheaply and still manage to eat low-fat meals, but this requires canny budgeting, and the knowledge of how to do this comes from education-based cultural capital.

The long history of hypocrisy of the upper-classes using some of the only enjoyments available to the working-classes/peasants—those of drinking, feasting and fucking—to demonize and condescend, is discussed by Silvia Federici in *Caliban and the Witch: Women, the Body and Primitive Accumulation* (2004) in terms of the carnivalesque pleasures of the Sabbat. For the Sabbat involved "[m]uch eating and drinking, surely a fantasy at a time when hunger was a common experience in Europe. (How revealing concerning the nature of class relations at the time of the witch-hunt, that dreams of roasted mutton and ale could be frowned upon by a well-fed, beef-eating bourgeoisie as signs of diabolical connivance!)" (Federici, 2004, p. 196). Such epicurean pleasures were practiced with discretion by the upper-classes because these goods were perpetually available to them, yet for the poor the feast was a break in the norm, coming *after* times of famine—and unsurprisingly with it came a breach of decorum, an unruliness of fleeting freedom that disturbs the *status quo* as a direct threat to the upper classes.

The pleasures of the carnival are described not just as epicurean in nature: they are also sensual and visceral, to do with the low realms of bodily functions that must therefore be repressed. It seems that even the feelings of disgust that such alimentary functions provoke have strongly classed dimensions. Bourdieu comments, "[D]isgust is the ambivalent experience of the horrible seduction of the disgusting and of enjoyment, which performs a sort of reduction to animality, corporeality, the belly and sex, that is, *to what is common and therefore vulgar*, removing any difference between those who resist with all their might and those who wallow in pleasure, who enjoy enjoyment." (2010, p. 491, italics mine). The connections between food, the body and vulgarity are made explicit in Elspeth Probyn's *Carnal Appetites: FoodSexIdentities,* where she comments: "In eating, pleasure offers itself to be problematized, as it brings our senses to life, it also forefronts the viscerality of life." (2000, p. 7). The pleasures of eating are close to the pleasures of sex geographically: the spaces of the body where food, sex, defecation, urination and orgasm take place are similar realms, blurring notions of inside and outside as well as proper and improper, polite and vulgar.

An endeavor to forge connections between the pleasures of sex and those of eating, is attempted by Probyn's book, but unfortunately ends up complicit in promoting the middle-class pleasures of exclusivity and rareness. The sensuality of eating is described using images of sex organs: Probyn describes an opening of a new "hip" Sydney restaurant that served "'Creaming Cock,' which compels the eater to go down on large tulle cones with apple-ginger custard and Tokay caramel ... The *piece de resistance* was ... the 'slice of pride,' a beautiful pink and white ice cream triangle, which, in true commensal fashion, we were asked to share." (Probyn, 2000, p. 65). The use of genitalia simulacra to signify "sexy" food feels rather reductive and superficial, although perhaps it might be delightfully amusing—*if* you could afford to eat at this restaurant. There is nothing here that speaks of the bodily experiences of the taste and texture, of *fullness*, the things that make eating sensual and pleasurable: instead it seems to use sex to sell sensual experience as a commodity for the bourgeois clientèle of a hip restaurant: as gimmick, and yet another way of acquiring cultural capital.

This *naughty but nice*, cleaned-up version of the murkiness of sensual pleasure of eating described by Probyn escapes its connection to the bodies which possess these carnal appetites. Which brings us back to the fleshy appetites of the corpulent body, and an analysis of the visceral flesh banquets on display at Jenny Saville's exhibition at Modern Art Oxford (23 June—16 September 2012).

The paintings were on a monumental scale, the figures looming large over the spectators. I found that the closer I got to the paintings, the more I lost a sense of the painted bodies' limits and boundaries, they became abstract when up-close, their borders bleeding out to form landscapes of flesh, colour and texture. In *Fulcrum* three women are laid-out upon each other horizontally as if served up on a banquet table; the masses of formless bodies form hilly flesh-tones, female mountains of corporeal geography. The paint so thick that it formed three-dimensional textures that rise up and away from the canvas, heavy, pregnant with the weight of all this paint. The fleshy abundance of *Fulcrum* makes it very difficult not to touch the multiple layers of surfaces in this painting. In an interview, Saville has said of this layering that: "I'm more interested in painting areas of flesh. It's as if the paint tends to become the body. It's like sculpture or something. When I put the paint in layers. It's like adding layers of flesh. There are areas of thick flesh, where the paint becomes more dense" (Saville in Sylvester, 2005, p. 14). This is the reverse of what is most commonly done to images of women, Saville is interested in putting back the flesh that is so often erased from women's bodies and in doing so demonstrates the sensuality inherent in our bodily corporeality and viscerality.[2]

Standing close to *Fulcrum*, I started to feel disorientated. I started off experiencing an aesthetic pleasure in gliding my eyes over such a visual feast, the drips, scratches, dabs and blobs of the paint. But as I took a step back, wanting to devour the whole composition, I began to lose any points of reference: where did one body start and another end? These interlocking bodies that seep and bleed into one another made me feel dizzy; the effect of bodily invasion stirred my stomach, making me feel disoriented and queasy as if from overindulgence.

What gives the corpulent body the aspect of visual terror is its presentation of bodies that have been othered by a society that is fearful of feminine corporeality. In *Volatile Bodies* Elizabeth Grosz suggests, "that women's corporeality is inscribed as a mode of seepage" (1994, p. 203). Taking up Julia Kristeva's theories of abjection (1984), and Mary Douglas's concept of dirt and taboo in *Purity and Danger* (1966), Grosz states of the sexual difference inherent in discourses around bodily excretions and viscous fluid that is treated as (fearfully) feminine: "[T]he horror of femininity, the voraciousness and indeterminacy of the vagina dentata [... is the] horror of subversion, the fear of being absorbed into something which has no boundaries of its own." (1994, p. 194). Grosz's suggestion is that we think, treat and end up experiencing human corporealities as gendered. She continues:

2 To see this image of Jenny Saville's Fulcrum please visit: http://www.saatchigallery.com/aipe/jenny_saville.hm.

> It is not the case that men's bodily fluids are regarded as polluting and contaminating for women in the same way or to the same extent as women's are for men. It is women and what men consider to be their inherent capacity for contagion, their draining, demanding bodily processes that have figured so strongly in cultural representations, and that have emerged so clearly as a problem for social control (Grosz, 1994, p. 197).

The corpulent body baulks at these pressures and rebels against the regulation of flesh on women's bodies as marks of excess, which through the normalization effects of airbrushing, surgery and diets can be reduced and disappeared. This supposed excess comes to be seen as bodily abjection: the excess flesh is felt not to belong to the body, but to be its "weight" and therefore its waste. What will be discussed now is how the "abject body" can be seen as subversive, a body that transgresses its own limits to flaunt its own corporeality.

The theory of abjection advanced by philosopher Julia Kristeva in *Powers of Horror* (1984) attempts to account for the fear *and* fascination we experience when encountering or thinking about our bodily fluids, viscera and waste, according to Kristeva, "It is not lack of cleanliness or health that causes abjection but what disturbs identity, system, order. What does not respect borders, positions, rules. The in-between, the ambiguous, the composite." (1984, p. 4). What is perhaps most revealing about Kristeva's theories of abjection is the way in which it describes the oppression of women through the disavowal of the very fact and function of their bodies. It is the very fecundity of the female body that is treated as horrifyingly abject: menstrual blood, breast milk, the moistness of the vagina and the dark unknown of the womb. In Saville's paintings the idea of bodily abjection is ever present as the abundant flesh also "disturbs identity, system, order" and "does not respect borders, positions": the masses of flesh endlessly unfold and reveal that which is usually hidden.

The argument that disgust can act as a form of knowledge-gathering, in that it prompts the viewer to make thought-inquiries about the state of bodies' representations in art history as well as in culture and society is taken up by Michelle Meager in her essay *Jenny Saville and A Feminist Aesthetics of Disgust* (2003). By making connections between disgust and an ethical encounter with the other, Meager argues that Saville's art of *unknown* bodies provokes knowledge of others' realities, suggesting that "Saville presents bodies rarely appreciated in contemporary Western culture. In a cultural climate that encourages women to conceal, if not exercise, those parts of their bodies considered fat, jiggly, out of control, and excessive, Saville insists upon revealing precisely these features" (Meager, 2003, pp. 23–41). Continuing the theme of physical disgust as visual and moral inquiry, she writes, "The fat female body, laid bare on Saville's canvas, provides an opportunity to find out what disgusts, and what disgusted and disgusting bodies can do, and in short it offers the opportunity to pay attention to the visceral reminders of how we embody social contexts and cultural expectations" (Meager, 2003, pp. 23–41). This idea of "visceral reminders" is a useful way of feeling-out transgression taking place, our tastes and value judgements are so ingrained as to become part of our body, and when seeing images that breach codes of good taste we often experience it physically in our gut, and in the example of the case studies presented here, this gut feeling is a sign something subversive is happening.

Speaking of her choice to use fat bodies in her work, Saville comments: "We live in a time where that type of body is abhorrent. A body this size represents excess, lack of control, going beyond the boundary of what's socially acceptable. I wanted the paint itself to be kind of obese, to have a diseased quality to the paint—an overabundance of paint on the surface" (Saville in Schama, 2005, p. 127). It is by making flesh that is so taboo the main focus of her work that Saville makes her paintings so viscerally disquieting. They are also portraits of flesh *itself*, presenting the excessive and culturally undesirable as worthy of regard, pleasure and appreciation.

The act of transgressing the rules of Western morality and art history—rules that posit that bodies categorized as "disgusting" or "bad taste" can only be experienced negatively as morally or physically unpleasant—can provide a source of subversive pleasure; for Georges Bataille, indeed, this transgression is the definition of eros. In *Eroticism* he asserts, "Because beauty counts insofar as ugliness cannot be further sullied, and the essence of eroticism is filth itself … Beauty is desired in order that it may be fouled; not for its own sake, but for the joy brought by the certainty of profaning it" (Bataille, 1987, p. 144). Bataille's assertion then is that there is a strong element of pleasure and delight in the embracing bad taste itself. Certainly one of the thrills of Saville's paintings is their nearness to yet deviation from traditional nudes, the flamboyant exposure of bodies that aren't classically beautiful in a setting in which we are expecting conventional beauty.

This also demonstrates the way a body thought of as ugly, or disgusting—not a body that is surface perfection and beauty, but a body that is a product and producer of abjection—shares an affinity with the murkiness of sexuality itself, as Carol Korsmeyer's writing confirms, "[D]isgust becomes part of deep aesthetic apprehension of difficult experiences, including some that might even qualify as beautiful—and even more surprisingly as delicious" (2011, p. 9). Therefore, the sexuality of the fat body can also spark a realization of the pleasures inherent in the reclamation of supposed "bad taste," alongside an inclusive approach to disgust and the viscerality that is vital to life. Through such reclamation we can reject shame to recast the fat body as an *agent provocateur* of feminist visual pleasure and subversive desire.

References

Bakhtin, M. (1984) *Rabelais and His World,* London, John Wiley & Sons.

Bataille, G. (1987) *Eroticism*, France, Marion Boyars Publishers Ltd.

Berlant, L. (2011) *Cruel Optimism*, London, I.B. Tauris.

Bordo, S. (1993) *Unbearable Weight, Feminism, Western Culture and The Body*, London, England, University of California.

Bourdieu, P. (2010) *Distinction: A Social Critique of the Judgement of Taste.* London, Routledge.

Deans, J. (2013) Jamie Oliver bemoans chips, cheese and giant TVs of modern-day poverty. *The Guardian.* Available at: http://www.theguardian.com/lifeandstyle/2013/aug/27/jamie-oliver-chips-cheese-modern-day-poverty.

Dury, S. and Thorp, S. (1994) *Viz, The Big Fat Slags Book*, John Brown Publishing.

Federici, S. (2004) *Caliban and the Witch: Women, the Body and Primitive Accumulation,* Brooklyn NY: Autonomedia.

Fielder, L. (1978) *Freaks: Myths and Images of the Secret Self*, Middlesex, England. Penguin Books.

Foucault, M. (1991) *Discipline and Punish: The Birth of the Prison*, London, Penguin Books.

Grosz, E. (1994) *Volatile Bodies: Toward a Corporeal Feminism*, USA, Indiana University Press.

Hartley, C. (2001) "Letting Ourselves Go: Making Room for the Fat Body in Feminist Scholarship," pp. 60–73, in *Bodies out of Bounds, Fatness and Transgression*, London, University of California Press.

Jones, O. (2011) *Chavs: The Demonisation of the Working-Class*, London, Verso.

Korsmeyer, C. (2011) *Savouring Disgust: The Foul and the Fair in Aesthetics*, Oxford, Oxford University Press.

Kristeva, J. (1984) *Powers of Horror: An Essay on Abjection*, Columbia University Press.

Lyons, P. (2009) *Prescription for Harm: Diet Industry Influence, Public Health Policy, and the "Obesity Epidemic"* pp. 75–87 in *The Fat Studies Reader*, eds. Rothblum, E., Solovay, S., New York and London, New York University Press.

Meager, M. (2003) "Jenny Saville and A Feminist Aesthetics of Disgust" *Hypatia* 18 (4) pp. 23–41 Fall/Winter 2003.

Orbach, S. (2009) *Bodies*, London, Profile Books.

Orbach, S. (1998), *Fat is Feminist Issue*, London, Arrow Books.

Probyn, E. (2000) *Carnal Appetites: FoodSexIdentities*, London, Routledge.

Schama, S. (2005) *Jenny Saville*, Rizzoli International Publications.

Skeggs, B. (1997) *Formations of Class and Gender: Becoming Respectable*, London, SAGE Publications Ltd.

Tyler, C.A. (2003) *Female Impersonation*, New York, Routledge.

Wann, M. (2009) in *The Fat Studies Reader*, eds. Rothblum, E., Solovay, S., New York and London, New York University Press..

Chapter 6
All Hail the Fierce Fat Femmes

Vikki Chalklin

> "Do we have any chubby people in the house?" The audience cheer. "Do we have any chubby fuckers in the house?" With a pout and a raised eyebrow, a round, besequined, and heavily made up man on stage takes a moment to carefully dab the sweat from his forehead with the glitter slash curtain behind him. "Chubby people, find those chubby fuckers. Let's lock the doors and we'll turn this into one big chase! I'm all for chub rub tonight ladies and gentlemen." (Scottee, *Hamburger Queen* 2013)

Hamburger Queen was a 'beauty pageant and talent show for fat people' (Scottee 2014a) run from 2011 to 2014 by London-based performance artist Scottee.[1] Scottee's work is brash, loud, and draggy, encompassing variety entertainment, avant-garde live art, and mainstream media.[2] His work has frequently dealt with issues around gay/queer identity, femininity, shame, food, and fat. *Hamburger Queen* was produced under the umbrella of the registered charity ScotteeInc., which works to develop community-minded art and performance projects using popular entertainment forms to engage people who don't feel included by the art world or think art is for them (Scottee 2014c). This annual performance event was framed as a competition in which self-identified fat people with a penchant for showing off were invited to compete to be crowned 'Queen' in front of a rowdy cabaret audience. Contestants competed in rounds with a panel of subcultural celebrity judges assessing their fashion sense, cooking skills, and performance talent. Yet this was no ordinary beauty pageant or talent contest. The organisers, judges, performers, and crowd were not interested in euphemistically 'curvy' beauties, a normative image of fashion sense, impressive performance skills, or even great cookery (many contestants brought intentionally disgusting, bizarrely decorated, or shop bought offerings for the 'taste' round). *Hamburger Queen* was an irreverent, camp, raucous, messy spectacle flying in the face of established discourses of both fat and LGBT politics that unapologetically dared the audience to take it seriously. In this chapter, I wish to position *Hamburger Queen* as a celebration of two embodied identities frequently

1 During 2011 and 2012, the event was known as Burger Queen until a legal battle forced the organisers to change the name to Hamburger Queen (Scottee 2014b).

2 For more information on Scottee's work, please see www.scottee.co.uk.

marginalised in both heteronormative and queer culture, namely femme and fat. I will do this through the methodology I have developed that I call performance autoethnography (Chalklin 2012), drawing together the value of performance as ethnographic object and method as proposed by Norman K. Denzin (1997, 2003), and the call for reflexive, located (auto)ethnographic practices argued for by Carolyn Ellis (2004) and rooted in the concerns of feminist epistemology (Haraway 1998, 2004; Stanley and Wise 1990) and queer theory (Halberstam 1998; Newton 1979, 2000; Delany 1999). Thus this chapter will primarily reflect upon my own experiences of *Hamburger Queen* as an audience member, and in the final 2014 competition, a contestant and finalist.

Part immersive performance art event-cum-installation and part showcase competition, *Hamburger Queen* was an ambiguous and very queer event that is not easily identifiable. The contest itself was, of course, the heart of the show. Three rounds took up the majority of the event – trend: flaunt your fatshion, talent: show off, and taste: serve something delicious to eat. Time between rounds was devoted to performances from a range of live artists and cabaret acts, video blogs relating to fatness and/or food, Scottee's hosting banter and progressively unpredictable interactions with the (increasingly inebriated) celebrity judges.[3] The event was, however, much more than this, and took its theme of a camp revisioning of retro Americana fast food aesthetics to the extreme. The venue (for all but 2014's final the infamous and historical gay cabaret and performance venue, the Royal Vauxhall Tavern) was decked out in formidable quantities of red and gold glitter slash fabric. The event had its own branding, theme tune, video idents and graphics to announce each round. Scottee, the co-host and head judge (for the first three years lesbian performer and organiser of legendary London performance club *Duckie*, Amy Lamé,[4] replaced by international plus-size model Felicity Hayward for the fourth and final year) and 'door whore'[5] Ginger Johnson were dressed in co-ordinated sequin burger joint uniforms,

3 Just some of the surprising judges' actions over the years include Lisa Stansfield giving an impromptu performance, June Brown (the actress portraying Dot Cotton in popular soap Eastenders) extolling the virtues of smoking to maintain a trim figure, and actor and comedian Matt Lucas leaving before the end of the event.

4 For more information on Duckie, please see www.duckie.co.uk. For an in-depth academic analysis of Duckie, alongside other London-based queer performance clubs, see Chalklin 2012.

5 'Door whore' is a colloquial term for the person stationed at the entrance to a club, bar, or performance event who collects entrance fees or tickets. This term is particularly commonly used in a tongue-in-cheek manner at queer clubs and cabaret events where this role is often carried out by elaborately dressed drag performers or people of ambiguous gender, becoming an integral part of the evening and making this activity a performance act in itself.

and a stall sold T-shirts, plastic hamburger handbags, and badges proclaiming 'Chubby' or 'Chaser'.

Whilst the reference to chubby chasers is cheeky, sassy, and brazen, this is not the dingy late-night-television portrayal of attraction to fatness as a freakish perversion or bizarre fetish. Fat bodies were the focal point at *Hamburger Queen* as they would parade, show off, strut and swagger, revelling in an admiration that is hard to come by in a fatphobic culture. Normative assumptions about fat being inherently undesirable were as conspicuously absent as the supposedly slimming voluminous sacks we are supposed to conceal our unsightly bodies beneath in the name of flattery. The campy parody of the beauty pageant format provided a platform for the contestants to plume and preen, exhibiting their bodies in any way they wished. In a glittering whirlwind of latex, fishnet, sequins and lace, the audience were invited to cheer, marvel, and appreciate undulating bare flesh and rolls of flab that in a world of fat shaming and hegemonic media glorification of thinness are rarely seen. For the contestants, *Hamburger Queen* was an opportunity to wear outfits that may be too outrageous, too skimpy, too sexy or too brash to wear out in public in any other circumstance. Myriad shades of fat femme-ininities indulged in gaudy flamboyance from gold lamé leggings to neon spandex body suits, lingerie to ball-gowns and corsets to cocktail dresses, with homespun costumes made from cuddly toys, cookery books, sweets, and cardboard cut-out sea creatures. The atmosphere was unmistakably carnivalesque, and once you stepped into this universe of flab and sequins, you realised the world had definitely been turned on its head.

No fats, no femmes

> I don't want to be put in front of a mirror by a stylist and called a piece of fruit and made to cry for the nation. I don't want to do that! I don't want to get my fat out for someone who can only be described as a Muscle Mary, on a television programme and be told that my body is embarrassing and fat.[6] Not interested. (Scottee, speaking at *Hamburger Queen* 2013)

> I just want to say that since I've started this competition I feel like I've changed so much and I've eat[en] for the first time without feeling guilty and … I'm just

6 This remark appears to be a reference to Dr. Christian Jessen, an out gay male television personality and medical doctor known for appearing in *Embarrassing Bodies* (2007), a reality series showcasing and treating the supposedly shameful medical ailments of the general public, and it's recent spin-off focused explicitly on 'obesity', *Embarrassing Fat Bodies* (2011).

going to embrace who I am from now on. (Ashleigh, on accepting the title of *Hamburger Queen* 2013)

The creation myth of *Hamburger Queen* tells of Scottee riding a London bus, frustrated and infuriated by the increasing normativity and body fascism rampant in a supposedly liberated gay culture now articulated around Grindr profiles with the common tagline 'no fats, no femmes' (Scottee 2014a).[7] Indeed, in a culture where 'obesity epidemic' rhetoric is ubiquitous and indisputable, *Hamburger Queen*'s unabashed celebration of chub is radical, and it is also, not coincidentally, incredibly queer. Primary themes throughout this short chapter are the crossovers between fat and queer that, through various guises, took centre stage at *Hamburger Queen*. Though the intersections between these identities have been explored in a number of academic and activist frameworks (Barker 2009, Bergman 2009, LeBesco 2004, Tovar 2012, Young 2013), they remain largely absent from mainstream fat acceptance discourse. Francis Ray White (2014) has argued that the role fatness plays in establishing and/or resisting or undermining binary gender legibility offers fruitful possibilities for a radical fat politics that could work to dismantle a range of normative binary distinctions. It is within this rich potentiality that I wish to place *Hamburger Queen*, as an example of fat activism that uses the camp trash aesthetics and ambiguous affect often favoured in queer modes of cultural production to dismantle all manner of normative discourses, including ones from within fat liberation and LGBTQ cultures. Bringing together two sites of normativity and marginalisation lurking in queer and fat activism, *Hamburger Queen* challenges and repudiates both the heteronormative and binary gendered bias in much dominant fat activism, and the invisibility and undervaluing of femme-ininities in various queer cultures.

Whilst the competition was open to anyone self-identifying as fat who wished to participate, the vast majority of contestants were feminine/femme presenting people, with a very high proportion of lesbian, gay, bisexual, or queer-identified participants. This may be due to a number of reasons, including the beauty pageant association perhaps being less likely to appeal to or resonate with masculine/butch presenting or identifying people, the rather differently manifesting social stigma around male fatness (see, for example, Barker 2009, Bergman 2009, Young 2013), or simply the high camp spectacle of the event. The reasons for this bias are not something I have the ability or inclination to examine here, but it does create the foundation for my key argument here, namely, that *Hamburger Queen* showcased, celebrated, and even enabled myriad shades of fat femme identification and embodiment. Fat women, queerness,

7 Grindr is a social networking app for smartphones aimed at gay and bisexual men that uses geolocation to provide users with a list of men by physical proximity, primarily to enable immediate sexual encounters.

and femme flair were unmistakably at the forefront of *Hamburger Queen*, making it a fat femme feminist carnival of camp in which norms, whether of gender, sexuality, or body size, were lampooned to the extent that they, even if only temporarily, disintegrated entirely. In an environment in which irreverence and glitter are the only conventions, queer femininity thrives.

> I'm huddled in a corridor behind a stage, hugging three women I barely know, all of us in in various states of undress. In our group hug, folds of naked flesh, rounded bellies and breasts squish together in a hot, sticky, cocktail of nerves and excitement. 'Chub love!' One of them sings. 'Break a leg fatsos!' I chime, and then suddenly the stage manager turns to one of them, nods, and she clambers up the three wooden steps that lead to the stage. In my sassy parody of a 1950s housewife, hair in rollers and a headscarf and wearing only lingerie and an elaborately kitsch apron made entirely of pictures of pin-up girls and cupcakes, my fatness and femmeness have never felt so constitutive of one another. Somehow, in real life, I always feel more visibly one or the other. Here, I don't have to lay the groundwork for any of it, I can just be my zaftig, queer, glittered and plumed self and nobody will bat a fucking false eyelash.

On 24th April 2014 I loudly and proudly proclaimed my fatness on stage at a sold out Bloomsbury Ballroom in West London, strutting my substantial stuff with three other fabulous fatties in the fight to be crowned the final ever *Hamburger Queen*. Having been introduced to fat activism, and through it, the emerging scholarly field of fat studies several years previously, to claim my fatness was not new to me, though it was unfamiliar and surprisingly powerful for me to do so in such a direct and unapologetically femme fashion. However, not all (and in fact, not very many) of the *Hamburger Queen* contestants were seasoned fat activists. For many, participating in *Hamburger Queen* was their first experience of body-positive space and rhetoric, and perhaps even of claiming the descriptor or identity of 'fat' for themselves. Moreover, for an audience largely composed of generally normatively sized fans of queer and cabaret performance, the body positive rhetoric of *Hamburger Queen* could be a revelation. Cat Pausé (2012) has utilised Goffman's (1963) theory of social stigma to examine the shame associated with fatness, and has suggested that 'coming out' as fat can be a powerful strategy for the management of this marginalised identity. Despite, in Goffman's terms, being a discredited (visually obvious and therefore not concealable) stigma, Pausé argues that fat can utilise the tactic from the gay and lesbian rights movement of emancipation through the (re)claiming of the stigmatised identity and vocabulary. In an anecdote about wearing a necklace displaying the word 'fat', she frames this tool of being 'out' as fat as powerful: 'I take pride in an act that feels delightful, subversive, but also mundane. This, for me, is what being out as fat is all about' (Pausé 2012: 52). *Hamburger Queen* was, as I have attempted to demonstrate above, far from mundane, though it was very much rooted in the everyday. In interviews about the show, Scottee repeatedly emphasised that the majority of contestants were not performers or activists, they were 'girls who work in call centres' (Scottee 2014b). The talent show/beauty pageant format also celebrated amateurishness – there was no expectation for the contestants to be skilled, experienced performers, bakers, or fashionistas, they were just meant to have fun.

As I will examine further in the next section of this chapter, the banter and rhetoric of *Hamburger Queen* also endlessly repeated the humdrum routine micro-aggressions fat people face on a daily basis, from flippant comments about diabetes and heart disease to ambivalent discussion of dieting and weight loss. There is a long tradition in fat activism and fat studies of working to identify, uncover, and critically analyse the mechanisms of normalisation through which fat people are routinely dehumanised in a hegemonic fatphobic culture, portrayed as 'a nebulous blob of people sometimes known as "the obese"' (Cooper 2010: 1024). Terminology such as 'the headless fatty' (Cooper 2007) has allowed scholars and activists to unpick the ways in which obesity epidemic discourse works to objectify fat people into a de-individualised, abhorrent and threatening mass. I would suggest that *Hamburger Queen* reacted to this de-individuation by staging a large-scale fat coming out. For the contestants, organisers, and potentially also a number of audience members, *Hamburger Queen* allowed for the proclaiming of fatness as a valid, valued, identity and/or aspect of embodiment. *Hamburger Queen* enacted the making visible of fat people not as faceless representatives of the 'Obesity Epidemic', but as individuals, on their own terms. For the contestants in particular, the showcasing of their personal sense of style, humour, culinary skill (or lack of), talents, tastes, interests, and voice became enmeshed with their fatness, as they were invited to perform a subjectivity of which fat embodiment is a valuable and constitutive part, not a shameful affliction or jibe.

Obstinate Fatties

Hamburger Queen operated from within a cultural context of 'obesity epidemic' rhetoric that incessantly characterises fatness (and by extension, fat people), as inherently morbid in more than just name. From tales of diabetes and heart disease, to the impending apocalypse of the 'obesity timebomb' and the burden they pose to public health systems, supposedly groaning under the weight of our increasing heft, fat people are positioned in the cultural imaginary as either killing society itself, or literally about to drop dead as a result of their fatness. Francis Ray White (2012) has insightfully examined this association of fatness with death, and the accompanying reach towards a more positive (slender) future through the theoretical framework provided by Lee Edelman (2004). Aside from some valid and insightful critiques of Edelman's work, White uses it to read anti-obesity rhetoric as exactly the kind of call to reproductive futurism Edelman takes issue with – we must do something about obesity, think of the children! If, like queers, fat people are already associated with the death drive as far as broader culture is concerned, White suggests perhaps we need to make like the problem we supposedly cause and embrace our ability to disrupt, challenge, and mess up the status quo of normative identities and bodies. This flies in the face of an increasingly potent propensity for a fat politics that hinges on healthism, specifically expressed through the paradigm of Health at Every Size (Cooper 2010). This focus on the need to disassociate fat from health, and highlight that many fat people are and can be perfectly healthy enacts what Kathleen LeBesco (2004) calls the 'will to innocence' (114) in fat politics. Whilst this attempt to position fat people as equally competent and therefore worthy may have its place, LeBesco and others have argued that this strategy simply works to limit an individual's responsibility for their own fatness, rather than working to challenge the very normative assumptions, ideologies, and frameworks of value and productivity fatphobia is based upon. Drawing on queer activist tools, LeBesco suggests a more powerful approach might come from the willful taking up of the problematic discourses that demonise fat bodies in order to corrupt and dismantle their moral power.

Hamburger Queen was dogged by problems resulting from the proximity of fatness and its pathologisation via 'obesity epidemic' rhetoric throughout its run – sponsors pulled out at the last minute, mainstream press refused to give it publicity, the organisers faced vicious Twitter attacks and even contestants regularly dropped out, all because of the perception that the show promoted 'obesity' and an unhealthy lifestyle, something many companies, journalists, broadcasters and individuals do not want to be seen to condone. Yet *Hamburger Queen* unashamedly and with a super-sized portion of irony and flippancy revelled in the discourse of the obesity epidemic – there was no recourse to how healthy or fit the contestants were, and while they were celebrated as beautiful, this is far from a normative or narrow definition of beauty. Whilst there have been contestants who employed the narrative of healthism, this was not central to the event itself, and it was their outrageous and brash swagger, rather than their claims of health and fitness, that were appreciated. Gourmet burgers were served, there were frequent jokes about diabetes and heart disease, and for the final run in 2014 Scottee commissioned an all-fat tap troupe called The Cholesterols to perform every week. However, *Hamburger Queen*'s raucous messy camping of 'obesity' discourse also resistsed dominant modes of fat liberation manifested through sincerity and earnestness. Murray (2008) has critiqued the dominance of what she calls 'feel good discourses' in fat acceptance movements that belie the power, cultural capital, and privilege behind the universal and uncritical call to 'love yourself'. In a critical move echoing the rejection by many queer scholars of gay pride politics and subsequent revaluing of negativity, shame, and trauma (Edelman 2004, Halberstam 2011, Halperin and Traub 2010), Murray suggests fat politics requires a similar complexity that is able to tolerate identities that are ambiguous, troubled, and shifting. One of the most interesting factors of *Hamburger Queen* is the way in which it made space for tensions, contradictions, and difficulties within fat activist discourse or fat acceptance space. One such tension placed centre stage in the 2013 competition is the issue of dieting, weight loss and gain, and how fat you have to be in order to be considered a fat activist. In 2012, drag queen contestant Ginger Johnson was criticised for being too thin to participate, and in recourse in 2013 took part in a segment where each week she would deliberately attempt to get fatter, being weighed in front of the audience in a nod both to the public weighing shame of slimming clubs and the problematic definition of how fat is fat, and in particular, how fat is fat enough to compete in a fat beauty pageant.

These ambiguous moments indicate how at *Hamburger Queen*, nothing was ever straightforwardly jovial or sincere, but rather intentionally ambivalent, always intertwining sincerity, gravity and parodic camp as a queer strategy of hybridity (Butt 2007). With roots in camp and a solid grounding in historic queer cultures, the 'queer kind of sincerity' (92) proposed by Gavin Butt in relation to queer and drag performance also serves as a useful tool for understanding the complex and ambiguous affective milieu created at *Hamburger Queen*. With its high camp aesthetic and flippant parodying of obesity epidemic discourse, *Hamburger Queen* employed irreverence as a mode of resistance to normative codes of seriousness that are pervasive in social movements. However, this burlesquing was not purely dismissive or frivolous to the exclusion of the serious questions it raises around stigma, pathologisation, and even health. A myriad of fat identities were showcased at *Hamburger Queen*, including the proud, joyous, fatty who may or may not be healthy, fit, or virtuous in their diet regardless of their size, the competent, confident, and able bodied, as well as disabled, debilitated, or traumatised fat people struggling with ill health, low self-confidence, or even attempted weight loss. The 'talent' round performances varied from high energy dance routines and cabaret acts with proudly jiggling flab, to heartfelt and heartbreaking performance poetry telling of rejection, trauma, shame, and marginalisation. In the 2013 season, Scottee and Amy Lamé took part in a weekly video series entitled *Why Are You Fat?* (2013) in which fat activist, scholar, former contestant and psychotherapist Dr. Charlotte Cooper discussed with each of them their struggles with dieting, compulsive eating, childhood trauma around food and their relationships with their mothers. The videos are candid, raw and make for moving and/or deeply uncomfortable viewing, particularly in the alcohol-fuelled rowdy cabaret atmosphere in which they were shown. At one screening a small group of audience members persistently laughed throughout. On her own blog, Cooper (2013) frames this incident in relation to the cultural expectation of fat people to be funny, or to resort to comedy as a strategy to combat prejudice. Whilst I agree with this reading, I would suggest that this response also speaks to the intentionally turbulent affective resonance of an event where the expected emotional response is often not clear – are you supposed to laugh or be offended when Scottee jokes that the special gourmet cro-nut burgers being served are likely to give you diabetes or a coronary? Is this woman's angry rant about being fetishised for having 'blowjob lips' but shunned in public by her lovers seeking empathy, approval, or a knowing smile? It seems to be all of the above.

Thus *Hamburger Queen* deliberately created a cocktail of ambiguous and contradictory affect in which joy, delight, excitement, misery, anger and indignation could co-exist, and this is exactly where its queer potential lies, in finding how 'we might *queerly prize* something in not taking it seriously' (Butt 2009: 92). Whilst much of what was staged at *Hamburger Queen* had a serious, heartfelt, or poignant undertone (whether of personal trauma or institutionalised stigma) glimmering through its glossy glitzy satire, the camp setting made it difficult to consider that any of it was meant to be taken entirely and straightforwardly in earnest. In a culture imbued with 'obesity epidemic' discourse so ubiquitous it seems utterly unchallengeable, it seems that perhaps the most radical thing *Hamburger Queen* did was ask its contestants and audience to be at once genuine and irreverent about their own bodies, identities, and even health. To return to White's (2012) assertions regarding fatness and the death drive, *Hamburger Queen*'s staging of problematic and troublesome encounters for its audience and contestants may be 'opening up the possibility of multiple queer futures for fat which, despite their apparent anti-sociality, may in fact offer some of us more of a life' (White: 15). If we accept White's suggestion that fatness is associated with the death drive, and thus that a fat politics engaged with this negativity is needed, it seems that *Hamburger Queen* might form a rich (pun intended) site of exploration, for it positively gorged on its critique of reproductive futurism.

Fat Femme-inism

It is the morning after I have won my heat and been entered into the final of *Hamburger Queen* 2014. Feeling proud, joyous, and a little smug, I meet a friend to excitedly retell and dissect the night before over lunch. Still glowing in my delight, I am walking home when I hear a man's voice holler at me from the open window of a parked car. "Hey baby, come here and give me some of that deliciousness". Ignoring the familiar catcall, I keep walking, and in the same breath the man's shout turns angry: "Lose some fucking weight". I ignore him again, and bolstered by the lingering glow of last night's admiration, laugh to

> myself. Heteropatriarchy and fatphobia restored. As long as it is for the sexual gratification of a (seemingly) straight man, my fat is just fine, even worthy of appreciation. But as soon as I refuse that positioning, that same fat poses a problem: suddenly my fatness is shameful, abject, takes up too much space, needs to be eliminated. A few steps further along the road, I wonder if I should have responded. I try to stand up to this type of street harassment as often as I feel able, even if it is just to demonstrate to the perpetrator that fat isn't an insult to me. But today, I am preoccupied, and more than a little hungover, and by the time I think about it, I am already a few feet away and it is too late. Maybe I should have fired back a witty retort. Maybe I should have snapped his picture to submit to *Smile, Sizeist*.[8] The irony of my failure to respond on this of all days is not lost on me. I feel the heavy responsibility to reach out, to create teachable moments, to educate and change ignorant people's minds. Does it make me less of a fat activist, or even less of a deserving finalist because I failed to stand up to this man when given the ideal opportunity? No. Because *Hamburger Queen* isn't about being the perfect activist who always does the right thing. *Hamburger Queen* is about being an amateur, messing up, having fun, and daring to take up space on your own terms, however you please.

Whilst I am arguing that *Hamburger Queen* created a wonderfully deviant, unruly carnival of queer fat acceptance, this was ephemeral, and I am not necessarily suggesting that it created significant lasting change outside of the event itself (though, as Ashleigh's comment above demonstrates, on an individual level it most certainly did). According to Bakhtin's (1984) influential analysis of the carnival's crucial role in feudal society, dominant power structures and codes of conduct were temporarily overthrown during carnival in order to maintain the equilibrium of normativity throughout the remainder of the year. This may, to some extent, be true of the radical upheaval of norms staged at *Hamburger Queen*, as the anecdote above demonstrates, but I also want to argue that the mere creation of that environment, even if only temporary and fated to disappear once the glitter has washed away, is reparative in forming a utopic vision for another possibility. The Bacchanalia of flesh and queer femininity enacted through this event is radical in the way it engages in a practice of world-

---

8 *Smile, Sizeist* is a tumblr page owned and managed by fat activist and photographer Substantia Jones, on which she encourages users to respond to fat phobic public harassment by taking photographs of the perpetrators, and sending these, along with the story of what happened, to her to be published on the page. Although potentially problematic in terms of consent, this is an interesting mode of everyday activism in the way it allows for the mundanity of everyday micro-aggressions resulting from fat embodiment to be shared and discussed, and in how it critically reframes the objectification and dehumanisation of fat people.

making. As argued by José Muñoz (1999) in relation to Latino/a performance, performance practices are able to inaugurate new world formations for oppressed or marginalised groups. Drawing from Richard Schechner's (1985) characterisation of performances of transportation and performances of transformation, Muñoz (1999) examines the oppositional worldviews and political possibilities enacted through minoritarian performance practices, and how they performatively bring these potentialities into being. Rather than simply being temporarily delivered into an alternative (fictional) world for the duration of the performance itself (as in performances of transportation), transformative performances produce that alternative mode of being as real – they performatively enact the change of which they speak. Though Schechner (1985) aligns transformation performance more with cultural rituals such as coming-of-age celebrations, Muñoz (1999) locates this process of oppositional world-making in queer and Latina performance practices that enact alternative realities and possibilities:

> [these] utopian impulses [are] made manifest by the performers, cultural workers, and activists who are *not* content to merely survive, but instead use the stuff of the 'real world' to remake [a] collective sense of 'worldness' through spectacles, performance, and willful enactments of the self for others. (200, original emphasis)

Hamburger Queen takes on, dismantles, and willfully mis-uses the rhetoric of the 'obesity epidemic' in order to create a carnival of corpulence: 'labour[ing] to make worlds – worlds of transformative politics and possibilities' (Muñoz: 195). It mined the personal, political, specific and universal, the joyous and the traumatic, to create not only an oppositional perspective or fictional utopia, but a very real alternative world in the space between 'good fatties' and 'bad fatties', laughter and tears, and between what is 'real' and what is performance.[9]

There is, however, another reason that I have chosen to recount this particular story here, one that connects to Scottee's call for 'chubby chasers' cited at the beginning of this chapter, which is the powerful space that *Hamburger Queen* created for both feminism and fat sexuality (and particularly, feminine presenting people's active sexuality on their own terms). Beneath the showbiz razzle dazzle of the show lies the desire to re-signify fat bodies as valuable, varied, but particularly, as sexual, and sexy. This was cheekily implied through the employment of the beauty pageant mode, but it was also reinforced through

9 There is insufficient space here to consider in depth the disruption of the audience/performer binary here, and how the disruption of this boundary, along with the ambivalent affective resonance and ambiguity over the event being a contest, showcase, or immersive performance event contribute to its world-making power.

other means: there were frequent references, in *Hamburger Queen's* signature ambivalent satire, to the fetishisation of fat bodies in both gay and straight culture in the form of bears, feeders, Big Beautiful Women and Fat Admirers, as well as the more colloquial Chubby Chasers. Though many of these kinks can be considered problematic and objectifying of fat bodies, contributing to the dehumanisation outlined above, they were presented at *Hamburger Queen* through the same parodic camping that it reproduced 'obesity epidemic' discourse, and so were at once framed as concepts that may resonate with some but are also not to be taken entirely seriously. Through calling upon the objectification and fetishisation of (particularly female) fat bodies, *Hamburger Queen* invites the sexual appreciation of fat people, fat women, fat femmes, as attractive and sexy, without being too saccharinely earnest or resorting to the stereotype of the jolly-yet-sexy fat girl. The contestant's contributions also often played on the stereotypes of fat women with voracious sexual appetites, through near-naked Samba dancing, bondage-inspired or dominatrix outfits, sexy burlesque acts, and an extraordinary number of sexual puns in the taste round contributions, from 'Power-Bottom Burgers' to 'Fanny Juice' and 'Cream Pies' meticulously decorated to resemble vaginas. Whilst contestants took a number of different approaches to their presentations, many featured some assertion of themselves as sexual beings. This is particularly interesting in relation to the female and femme-focused nature of the environment, as fat women are in a cultural double bind of at once being shamed and denigrated as (and for) not being sexually attractive due to their fat, whilst women in general are positioned as having a sexuality that exists for the sole satisfaction of men, facing the label of slut if they do demonstrate a sexual appetite of their own. Add to this the further undervaluing of femme-ininities and disparaging of femme sexuality in many queer and lesbian spaces, and the creation of an environment in which fat, queer, femme women can claim and perform their sexuality on their own terms, and do so centre-stage whilst gaining unconditional appreciation for doing so seems impossibly utopian. To draw the discussion of world-making above into dialogue with José Muñoz's (2009) later work on queer futurity, I would suggest *Hamburger Queen* might be exactly one the things Muñoz is calling for when he evokes:

> an insistence on something else, something better, something dawning … necessary modes of stepping out of this place and time to something fuller, vaster, more sensual, brighter. (189)

As discussed above, White (2012) has suggested that 'obesity epidemic' rhetoric has already relegated the fat body from any kind of future in the linear 'straight' time Muñoz wants to leave behind, so it seems *Hamburger Queen* must exist in a parallel temporality that could be nothing but queer. You certainly can't get much 'fuller, vaster, more sensual, brighter' than the flesh, colour, and glitter slash of *Hamburger Queen*.

References

Bakhtin, M. (1984) *Rabelais and his World*, Bloomington: Indiana University Press.

Barker, J. E. (2009) 'Transfatty', in Tomrley, C., and Kaloski Naylor, A. (eds) *Fat Studies in the UK*. York: Raw Nerve Books, 32–34.

Bergman, S. B. (2009) 'Part-Time Fatso' in: Rothblum, E., and Solovay, S. (eds) *The Fat Studies Reader*, New York: New York University Press, 139–142.

Butt, G. (2007) 'How I Died for Kiki and Herb' in Rogers, H., ed. *The Art of Queering in Art*, Birmingham: Article Press, 85–94.

Butt, G. (2009) 'Should We Take Performance Seriously?' in Ashery, O., ed. *Dancing with Men*, London: Live Art Development Agency, 78–92.

Cooper, C. (2007) Headless Fatties [Online]. London. Available: http://charlottecooper.net/publishing/digital/headless-fatties-01–07 [Accessed 19/06/14].

Cooper, C. (2010) 'Fat Studies: Mapping the Field' *Sociology Compass*, 4:12, 1020–1034.

Cooper, C. (2013) Why do you laugh at fat people? [Online]. London. Available: http://obesitytimebomb.blogspot.co.uk/2013/03/why-do-you-laugh-at-fat-people.html [Accessed 19/06/14].

Delany, S. (1999) *Times Square Red, Times Square Blue*, New York: New York University Press.

Denzin, N. K. (1997) *Interpretive Ethnography: Ethnographic Practices for the 21st Century*, London: Sage.

Denzin, N. K. (2003) *Performance Ethnography*, London: Sage.

Edelman, L. (2004) *No Future: Queer Theory and the Death Drive*, Durham: Duke University Press.

Embarrassing Bodies (2007) [Television series] Channel 4. Maverick UK.

Embarrassing Fat Bodies (2011) [Television series] Channel 4. Maverick UK.

Ellis, C. (2004) *The Ethnographic I: A Methodological Novel about Autoethnography*, Oxford: AltaMira Press.

Goffman, E. (1963) *Stigma: Notes on the Management of a Spoiled Identity*. Englewood Cliffs, NJ: Prentice-Hall.

Halberstam, J. (1998) *Female Masculinity*, Durham: Duke University Press.

Halberstam, J. (2011) *The Queer Art of Failure*, London: Duke University Press.

Halperin, D. M. and Traub, V., eds. (2010) *Gay Shame*, Chicago: University of Chicago Press.

Haraway, D. (1988) 'Situated Knowledges: The Science Question in Feminism and the Privilege of Partial Perspective', *Feminist Studies*, 14(3), 575–599.

Haraway, D. (2004) 'A Manifesto for Cyborgs: Science, Technology, and Socialist Feminism in the 1980s' in Haraway, D., ed. *The Haraway Reader*, London: Routledge, 7–45.

Jones, S. (2013) Smile, Sizeist. [Website] Available: http://smilesizeist.tumblr.com [Accessed 19/06/14].

LeBesco, K. (2004) *Revolting Bodies: The Struggle to Redefine Fat Identity*, Boston: University of Massachusetts Press.

Muñoz, J. E. (1999) *Disidentifications: Queers of Colour and the Performance of Politics*, Minneapolis: University of Minnesota Press.

Muñoz, J. E. (2009) *Cruising Utopia: The Then and There of Queer Futurity*, New York: New York University Press.

Murray, S. (2008) *The 'Fat' Female Body*, Basingstoke: Palgrave.

Newton, E. (1979) *Mother Camp: Female Impersonators in America*, Chicago: University of Chicago Press.

Newton, E. (2000) *Margaret Mead Made Me Gay: Personal Essays, Public Ideas*, Durham: Duke University Press.

Pausé, C. (2012) 'Live to Tell: Coming Out as Fat' *Somatechnics*, 2:1, 42–56.

Schechner, R. (1985) *Between Theater and Anthropology*, Philadelphia: University of Pennsylvania Press.

Scottee (2014a) Happy Fatties are Erased from the Media [Online] Available: http://www.feministtimes.com/happy-fatties-are-erased-from-the-media/ [Accessed 19/06/14].

Scottee (2014b) Profile: Hamburger Queen [Online] Available: http://www.feministtimes.com/profile-hamburger-queen/ [Accessed 19/06/14].

Scottee (2014c) ScotteInc. [Web] Available: http://www.scottee.co.uk/#!inc/sitepage_3 [Accessed 19/06/14].

Stanley, L. and Wise, S. (1990) 'Method, methodology and epistemology in feminist research processes' in Stanley, L., ed. *Feminist Praxis: Research, Theory and Epistemology in Feminist Sociology*, London: Routledge, 20–60.

Tovar, V. (2012) *Hot and Heavy: Fierce Fat Girls on Life, Love and Fashion.* Berkeley, California: Seal Press.

White, F. R. (2012) 'Fat, Queer, Dead: "Obesity" and the Death Drive' *Somatechnics*, 2:1, 1–17.

White, F. R. (2014) 'Fat/Trans: Queering the Activist Body' *Fat Studies: An Interdisciplinary Journal of Body Weight and Society*, 3:2, 86–100.

Why Are You Fat? (2013) [Online video] Scottee. Available: https://www.youtube.com/watch?v=51vj64OA3qs [Accessed 19/06/14].

Young, M. (2013) Male Privilege and Transitioning From a Fat Woman to a Fat Man. *The Rainbow Hub* [Online]. Available: http://www.therainbowhub.com/male-privilege-and-transitioning-from-a-fat-woman-to-a-fat-man/ [Accessed 19/06/14].

Creative Interlude

Chapter 7

Hidden and Forbidden: Alter Egos, Invisibility Cloaks and Psychic Fat Suits

Jennifer Lee

In my writing I've always been driven to peel back the layers and reveal what is shameful or taboo in Western culture. Part of this process is to trigger questions for the reader, including: is this how you assumed life would or should be? What can you learn about your relationship to the world from facing what you are afraid of? There is value in examining what makes us uncomfortable about our lives, and the lives of others. My writing is often considered dark or disturbing, and I know that much of that perception is related to my exploration of the gendered body in sexual and taboo ways. This has ranged from writing about female paedophiles and serial killers (Lee, 2007) to transgender superheroes (Lee, 2013) and intersex characters.

During the writing process, partially submerged images, thoughts and feelings arise, and at times, disparate connections emerge. A teacher and writer who was pivotal to my development as a writer, Professor Kevin Brophy, encouraged me to allow these connections to occur in my writing without always understanding why they were bubbling up together. Later in the writing process, the connections often loop in interesting ways, or give another dimension to a piece. Brophy states in his book *Creativity: psychoanalysis, surrealism and creative writing*: 'Literature and the writing we call creative is risky: it involves exposing oneself as a writer to what is emotional and personal… ' (1998, p. 193).

These two notions – to allow disparate connections to emerge, and to tell risky stories in order to question aspects of my life – are the foundations of this chapter. The questions that arose as I reflected on my experiences are in some ways separate and in other ways intrinsically linked, and they often interact with further questions and pieces of narrative from my life. This chapter could be seen as an autoethnographic dance around the themes of fat, masculinities, sex and sexuality.

How did I feel both boyish and fat as a teen?

In high school I felt disconnected from the other girls. When they spoke about hair and make-up I remained silent. I wore my hair short and professed no interest in girly frivolities. When they revealed their crushes, I held mine in a shame-filled embrace. Shame because I felt that those boys were too good for boring, nerdy, chubby me. What did it mean to be an A+ Physics and advanced Maths student with only one or two other girls in those classes, where the boy you have a crush on wants your help in Maths and therefore cannot see you as a potential girlfriend because he would have to consider himself smarter at a traditional male field than you, in order to date you?

In my teen years, and into my early 20s, my sexuality felt masculine and I often saw it as a negative and secretive force in my life. As a teen I would sneak into the back room when everyone was asleep, turn on the video player and fast forward to find the sex scenes in my dad's foreign films. I identified with the men in the scenes, and in fact I had an accidental orgasm (while I rode a pile of pillows) before I knew what the word meant. I was about 10 years old and I thought, 'Do other people know about this?' Later, during Divinity classes at school, I learnt that this is masturbation and it is not allowed for strict Anglicans because it's sinful. But I couldn't resist. Through my teen years I drew naked stick figures having sex and masturbated to these pictures (it was the 80s, there was no Internet, and porn was harder to come by). I would then rip the pictures into tiny pieces and say a prayer asking God for forgiveness. The strangely looping prayer went: 'Dear God, please forgive me for masturbating. I can't promise I won't do it again, but I can promise I'll be sorry and pray for forgiveness each time'.

During this time I also believed I was fat and I preferred to use it as an invisibility cloak. By that I mean that my perceived fatness led to my assumption that no boys would be interested in me, and that was a safe option. Upon reflection I think the boys weren't interested in me because I suffered from anxiety and depression from a young age and barely spoke. The photos reveal that I was a fairly 'normal' size – not fat, not thin, but a teen with rounded edges.

Why did I dream of femme but sleep with butch?

When I first kissed a girl I was 20. She was my best friend. She had short hair, wore steel-capped Doc Martens boots and men's Bonds[1] t-shirts. She rolled her own cigarettes, drank pots of beer and only spoke to a few people. She was poorer than me so I bought her drinks. My lesbian writing teacher assumed I

1 Bonds is an iconic affordable Australian brand known for simple casual clothes.

was also a lesbian when I took Kate to a reading event and bought her beer. We went everywhere together – no one issued an invite to me without including her. But in terms of a physical connection, one drunken kiss is all we had – we were strangely in tune in some ways but not in others. She was a mean reckless drunk and gave her boyfriend a bloody nose several times. I spoke to her about hitting her boyfriend and she justified herself. She argued that violence was different when it came from women. With my zero tolerance for violence, and low tolerance for people who won't take responsibility for their actions, this was the tipping point of an already fractious relationship and I decided I couldn't handle the friendship anymore.

At that time I fantasised about tying up my flatmate's sociopathic but cute-and-girly-as-a-button girlfriend and sadistically topping her. I intensely disliked her in our everyday interactions – her values were far from mine. Instead of further exploring my attraction to women I pushed it into a corner of myself and labelled it, 'One day I might want to experiment and sleep with a woman but I only feel relationship-oriented towards men'. I then spent three years living with a boyfriend, Scott, who loved my body, even when I stopped dieting and put on 30 kilograms. I also spent those years having sexually violent nightmares.

When I said 'my writing is queer but I'm straight', did alarm bells ring?

I'd just started researching and writing towards a PhD in creative writing. I was researching intersex, masculinity in women and how gender roles are reinforced in our culture. These creative writing PhDs in Australia usually involve research in the cultural, social, gender or literary studies fields and culminate in a two-part thesis, a creative work such as a novel, and a theoretical work (an exegesis) that positions the creative work within a body of research.

My research sparks began with my gender-bending dreams and nightmares. The research then broadened to focus on the medical management of intersex births; representations of intersex characters and butch women in mainstream film, television and writing; and the symbiotic relationship between creative writing, life and dreams. When I began this research I was fat and a closeted queer. I had broken up my first long-term relationship with Scott in the suburbs and moved into an inner-city one-bedroom flat in Melbourne to live alone for the first time. It was some time after this, while researching intersex, when I met Jane and the notion of being a queer writer yet a straight woman started to crumble.

The process of coming out to myself happened in a cascade of epiphanies, all stemming from Jane touching my arm. At first, as I openly admitted to myself that I desire women, I was flooded with lust and I had no sexual interest in men for about six months so I began to call myself a lesbian. I said to a friend, 'I don't think I'll ever go back to men now'. Then, as the flood dissipated, I acknowledged that I still desired men so I began to come out as bisexual. I found these public declarations embarrassing because the various announcements of changing identity seemed to demonstrate a lack of self-knowledge. On top of this, as Jane's gender identity shifted outside the binary, and as my research into intersexed identities progressed, I began to dislike 'bisexual' as a term that divided the sexes into two. In fact, I 'came out' multiple times as I understood myself better yet I never really enjoyed the declaration of a permanent (new) identity.

In the end I wasn't sure what to call myself so I simplified things and just went with the broad term 'queer'. I am more comfortable with the umbrella term, and it captures bent sexuality and other non-normative sexual practices as well. I began to accept myself as a queer woman and a queer writer who writes about sex and gender. Fiona McGregor wrote about this uncovering of the self in her essay 'I am not a lesbian', and this quotation, while almost 20 years old, has always resonated with me:

> I think if you're placed on the margins of a society by being queer you have a head start in being perverse, and if you're perverse you have a head start in understanding more deeply the foibles and mysteries of human behaviour. It stands to reason that lives in an outer circle will to some extent revolve around those in the inner circle, but not the other way around. Social mores are the uniform on the body of human behaviour, and when one is disrobed, willingly or unwillingly, one uncovers what lurks beneath (1996, pp. 38–39).

In terms of what lurks beneath, there is a line in experienced mindfulness practitioner, Jon Kabat-Zinn's, meditation: 'Whatever it is, it's already here: let me feel it' (2007). It's a mantra of mine now, and I take it to mean – if there is something brushing at the edges of your conscious mind, troubling you, disrupting your life, you can try to repress it, but whatever it is, it's already here. Acknowledge it, bring it into the light, examine it, and if your life changes as a result, that's cleaner than the rotting self-deceit that hides beneath. Perhaps this is not something that everyone experiences, but those of us who have faced ourselves and come out – as queer or fat-embracing – I suspect understand this concept.

Did masculinity represent power to me?

Before I came out to myself in my mid-20s I had what I'll call Classic Freudian Repression Nightmares about raping feminine girls with a giant penis. I thought my head was sabotaging itself with nightmares that stayed with me all day.

I worked one of these dreams into the draft of the creative component of my PhD. The interplay between sex, masculinity and gender is a common theme in my dreams and my writing. Here is an edited version of that fictionalised dream:

> Justin slides his cock inside me and it melts into my flesh and fills me and smoothes my scars. I pull away from him and his shaft stretches between us like an elastic band. We play tug of war and I win, because I want it more than he does. The base becomes thinner until I pinch it off. I fly backwards and land on the bed. I rearrange the flesh like a kid with a strip of playdough. I stand up and push him onto the bed and stare at the place where his cock used to be. I push on his flesh and when I take my finger away, there is an indent. He has turned into a woman, with hair to her waist, straight and black. Her chest sprouts breasts and I place three fingers on the place where her cunt should be.
>
> I am sticking three fingers inside her and scooping her out, each scoop yanking a growl from the pit of her womb. I'm flicking her clit to the beat of her breath and licking her nipple – the invisible string of desire pulling her teat till it's hard and protruding. I kiss her as an animal devours meat, raw and bloody, all teeth and tongue. My cock grows longer the closer I get to coming.
>
> Flesh slips away to reveal two penises, nestled into her chest. They are contained within a sac. My fingernails tear open the hole and the cocks squeeze through the sac opening. I suck her right penis. The cocks become engorged, and one ejaculates into my mouth, one across my face. I come with no warning. I stand over her, and blood spurts out of my cock across her body. I watch my cock grow until it is a metre long. I look down at my breasts. They are bound with bandages; blood seeps through my top. I leave her lying there and launch into the air. I fly away, with my cock dripping semen over the city (2006, p. 120).

Embedded within this dream is a degree of body hatred and disgust, as well as a wish for a malleable body that can be transformed to fulfil forbidden desires. The dream also constructs a heterosexual binary sexuality but this shifts with imagery such as penises being torn from amniotic sacs. Dreams, and fiction inspired by or derived from dreams, have offered me a way to explore gender and the body and raise questions about our perceptions of binaries, without pinning down singular meanings.

How did I go from rejection of the feminine to identifying as a femme?

Because I had often felt masculine as I grew up, the expression or performance of femininity had always felt false to me. I then met a slim and androgynous Australian writer with a Chinese familial background. Jane had short black hair, and she wore faded blue Bonds[2] t-shirts. She was often told off in women's toilets when other women assumed she was male. I wore skirts around her but at first I feared she wouldn't like me unless I was more butch. But by then I had embraced long hair, make-up and heels and re-embraced dieting. I was 'curvy' at the time (thin for me) and perhaps that was why I had started to embrace the trappings of femininity, albeit with leather straps, buckles and bold jewellery.

In typical Australian style, the men don't ask the women out, even when the women make it really obvious they're open to it. Couples edge around each other until they're both drunk, and then they hook up. We did it a bit differently because I was supposedly straight, and because she was in a long-term lesbian relationship. We met for lunches and emailed late at night, until I felt that it was unethical not to declare my feelings, as feelings were developing, her relationship aside. After she broke things off with her partner, we started seeing each other.

While I had started to believe it is best to leave politics at the bedroom door, I'm not sure if I allowed myself to admit attraction to femme women at the time. I'm uncertain about whether I needed to reinforce myself as feminine, and a female partner who inhabited a masculine appearance and behaviours supplied a contrast for me, and allowed me the space to more fully express traditional feminine traits. At that time I wore a lot of heels, strappy sandals, skirts and red lipstick and lamented that I had to keep my fingernails short to protect sensitive spots. My vulnerability and sensitivity – often seen as female traits – also seemed heightened.

It was around this time that Jane and I went together to my friend's alter ego dress-up party. I dressed in tight pink and a short skirt, wore rabbit ears and voila! I was a Playboy bunny. A fat Playboy bunny in pink, a colour I've detested for a long time, probably because it represents (for me) the conditioning of little girls into traditional roles. Jane decided her alter ego was a man and she dressed as Tom of Finland, the queer visual artist: moustache, leather and socks down her pants. Actually I can't remember if it was socks but there was a definite bulge. We were an interesting looking pair. I went as the supposed straight man's fantasy girl, though fatter, and my girlfriend went as a bent gay man on the edges of edgy culture. I suppose you could see me trying to say, 'Look, I'm not *that* out there – there is a part of me that isn't a die-hard feminist who won't accept drinks from men at bars because I don't like power imbalance in everyday interactions'. And perhaps Jane was saying, 'I don't really want to conform to my current gender identity – I'm queerer than you think'.

In fact, soon after this party Jane asked me to call her James and use male pronouns in private, which I did. In public he remained Jane and used female pronouns, but in private he was James. Eventually he spent a few weeks coming

2 The blue Bonds t-shirt is particularly associated with working-class men in Australia.

out, and asked people to use male pronouns. I'm still not sure if he needed to try the different identity on in private for a while, with me, to reinforce that it was right, before declaring it publically, or if he needed to take the time to gather the strength for such a huge declaration. Perhaps both, but I don't profess to know. It seems understandable, if fractured, that his public-private gender presentation was different for a period of time.

Am I a woman that yields or wields?

I had fantasised about being dominated in the bedroom for a long time. Restrained, reprimanded, punished. I think the letting go of control appealed as much as the fun of embodying a traditional female role – submissive to a man or masculine figure – that denied self that I couldn't bring myself to embody in my everyday life. And that feminine self that I thought I failed to embody as a young girl with pageboy home haircuts and a teenager with short hair and clothes that hid my budding breasts. Yet in my fantasies of femme women I always cast myself as the top, in total control, and usually wielding a cock.

I'm not sure why my last crush was on my first femmy woman – a lipstick wearing, long-haired woman, albeit a feminist. I have a feeling it's to do with my practice of acceptance, which I have focused on in terms of being fat in recent years. This acceptance of the self has allowed me to shed the dichotomies and embrace the spaces in-between, which includes allowing my fantasies of femme women to co-exist with myself as I am (not a masculine version of myself with a giant penis).

As I have settled into my fat body and given up dieting (meaning I have also given up temporary states of relative thinness), I have found that heels are too uncomfortable for me to carry my fat body on so I've given them up too. And I don't miss them at all. I also wear less make-up because I commit the time to other things. By learning to accept my emotions rather than trying to control them, I overflow less often than I used to. Acceptance, emerging from my practice in fat and body acceptance, has also allowed me to develop a more complex (and less vigilant) view of my own gender identity and performance.

Was my bad body image because I was fat?

I feel that my view of my fatness limited my sex life for many years. I couldn't conceive of stripping for a man when at my fattest but even in those diet-induced periods of slimness – Australian size 14–16, which is still considered a bit porky – I wore a psychic fat suit. Because of course my feelings about my body didn't change just because I lost weight. At 130kg, just after a break-up,

I travelled to Thailand and several Thai men who seemed fascinated by my body pursued me. One didn't speak English but drew love hearts in the palm of my hand. I was shy and not used to the idea of sex with no intellectual or emotional connection, which there couldn't be with the language divide. I also needed the safety of a relationship – reeling them in emotionally – before I could contemplate stripping. I needed to know they were in too deep to reject me based on my fat body. I think I assumed a potential partner would be disappointed in my body but think, 'Oh well, I really like her, so I'll overlook her bad body'.

My intermittent weight loss was primarily an attempt to feel attractive and attract men. An IT tech that helped me set up my internet over the phone liked the sound of me and wanted to meet up but I refused because I assumed he'd imagined a slim girl and I didn't want to see the look of disappointment on his face. In my brief experiences with Internet dating I always ticked the 'overweight' box and put up a realistic (password restricted) photo of myself – who wants to see a look of disappointment when they meet someone? I waged war on my body again as I began dieting and banning foods (like take-away, cheese and butter). I temporarily lost 30 kilograms and gained confidence (confidence that a culture that worships thin women, and therefore all men, would reject me less).

As I grew up, my father often critiqued my mother's body and told her she needed to lose weight. He also watched what my sister and I ate and told us when we didn't earn the food or if our serve was too large. That coupled with the slapping, hitting, punching and judgement of our bodies throughout puberty, and it was a recipe for shame and internalised fat hate. A friend of mine in my 20s tried to reassure me, 'If someone wants to sleep with you, they can tell what kind of body you have through your clothes. It's not like you'll undress and they'll be in complete shock about your body'. I was doubtful, as fat nakedness was, and still is, so absent from our culture. And I think I fooled myself into thinking that some control top pants and cleverly draped material could hide more fat than it did.

Why did accepting fat mean a grieving period for me?

Accepting my fatness meant accepting that I'd never conform to the ideal version of a feminine woman in our culture. Refusing a free drink from a man in a bar, not flirting or acting vulnerable or subjugating my intellect, and instead wanting to meet potential partners on equal ground, was not attractive to the majority of men I met, whether I was fat or thin. I think this was because it threatened their brand of vulnerable masculinity, hard to attain and maintain, based on being in a position to earn more (pay for drinks) or be taller or stronger or more reticent. I'm not bubbly or particularly good at small talk. Direct and observant, yet ready to argue a point, are considered more masculine traits in our culture. Those traits combined with being fat, and I couldn't be a vulnerable, light, submissive woman. Many women wouldn't consider themselves submissive to patriarchal culture but there are ways that I am (arguably annoying and time consuming hair removal) and ways that many women are. Questioning the gender assumptions that make us men and women is part of questioning what it means to be fat.

Having said that, I always lamented that I couldn't be the kind of woman who could be lifted and fucked against a wall or in the shower, although I'm sure a body builder could hold me up. Maybe my tendency to choose partners, male and female, who are unsporty intellectuals with little upper body strength, is part of the issue here.

Those montages in romantic comedies like *Going the Distance* (Burstein, 2010), where Justin Long lifts Drew Barrymore and carries her into the ocean, always give me a pang – because my fat body doesn't allow for that. I'll never be carried over a threshold after being married. The embarrassing fact that I secretly lament these traditional feminine moments that don't easily apply to a fat woman is incongruous with my rep as a feminist queer woman who wears a lot of black, boots, zips and jewellery with knives through hearts. The embarrassing (but now embraced) fact is that I love well-written romcoms that nevertheless mostly reinforce fantasy-perfect heterosexual relationships: *While You Were Sleeping* (Turteltaub, 1995), *When Harry Met Sally* (Reiner, 1989), even the politically unforgivable *Pretty Woman* (Marshall, 1990). In many ways I have always been looking for the romcom story – two people live happily ever after in a long-term relationship or marriage, with the implied future being children, a house, a dog, lovely holidays and harmony. My own parents had a house, a fractious dysfunctional relationship, children, no pet, and holidays filled with fights. And my mum asked my dad to marry her. Clearly, I wanted an upgraded version of my own upbringing. But I worked against those traditional values at times in my life – observing what they could lead to. So after I was incredibly hurt by two relationships ending in succession, I declared to my friends that I was going to have a fling.

Did I choose a fat fling to avoid rejection?

I wanted some more notches on my belt, perhaps to further prove to some inner subconscious critic that I was not the nice little frigid nerdy Christian all the kids at high school treated me as. I met up with a lesbian couple I knew and went to a queer porn launch in a warehouse with bad cask wine on sale for $2. It was perfect.

Across the room I locked eyes with a handsome man: dark haired with a Sri Lankan background. At the time I saw Craig as large – perhaps big-boned – but later I saw that he was fat. I had never slept with a fat person. I don't remember much about his fat that changed the actual sex, perhaps only my comfort levels with stripping for a fellow fatty. He was heavier on me and that was okay. I liked his substance – he was grabable and stronger than other sexual partners. But as I write this I think, his fat is a side note to the whole experience. I know that fat bodies are more significant to people who particularly desire them, or who are anti-fat.

Craig was bisexual – the first person I'd slept with who also desired more than one gender – and for the first time I was confronted with someone who was way less vanilla[3] than me. I said I was into s&m and I found myself being spat on (I didn't really care and wasn't offended but it was a turn off and I said so), and slapped and bruised (which was okay but not that satisfying – I realised later because I had no emotional connection with him), but the real challenge was what he told me he'd tried and wanted to try. Tried: drugs up the butt, group sex, watersports. Hoped to try: more bodily fluids including vomit, feederism[4] (which I'd never heard of) and animal-friendly bestiality. To all of which I gave a polite 'not even if the world was ending' response.

One morning after he stayed over he planted a magazine on the breakfast table as I served the eggs. I glanced down and saw the back of a chubby girl, wearing only white granny pants, with clumps of shit hanging in the back of her undies, which were stained brown. My response later prompted a good friend of mine to say, 'You are not judgmental enough. Sometimes judging people is okay'. I don't agree in this case and I stand by my decision to kindly remove the magazine from the table top and say, 'I'm sorry, that's not for me. There are places we crossover but that is not one of them'. Then, often the mollifier and conciliator, I offered to pee on him (but not to be peed on). We never got that far because, as I said to the same friend, 'It all feels so empty'. She gave an exasperated sigh and said, 'Jenny, it's a fling; it's not supposed to be the love of your life. You need to end it though because he doesn't seem to know it's a fling!' She was right, and I did. Less mature then, I cried because I felt guilty but I told Craig it was because I wasn't ready for a relationship. He asked for two more slices of toast, which I made for him before I sent him on his way.

3 'Vanilla' refers to sex that is not kinky or adventurous. This might vary from culture to culture. In western culture it implies no role play, toys, extra people, bondage, and so on. It most likely takes place in a bed.

4 Craig explained that feederism or feedism is the eroticisation of weight gain through eating food. I said I wasn't interested in being a feedee or gainer because it didn't turn me on, not because there was any judgement.

My friends assumed I broke it off because he was too sexually 'perverted' but it wasn't that. We didn't connect emotionally or intellectually and he didn't impress me. All my other partners had been, and have been since, impressive, intellectual, well-read, and people I feel proud to introduce at a party for those reasons. I have questioned if that is classist or status-oriented, and perhaps it is, because it goes beyond the connection you have with someone when you discuss similar interests and into territory about what status your partner has in the cultural circles in which you move. However, the thinness or fatness of a woman changes her status as well as her partner's status in any class in which they move, within Western culture. A fat woman paired with a traditionally handsome man will raise eyebrows – perhaps he is stupid? A thin woman paired with a fat man will matter less – I think it is assumed that he must be powerful or rich.

Perhaps as someone brought up to achieve – I have a strong memory of my father seeing my 98 per cent score on a Maths test and saying, 'Right, let's have a look at where you went wrong' – it is more difficult to accept how you fall short in the areas that our culture values most. I feel a sense of pride when I look over my queer sex history – that I'm not 'vanilla', that I explore my sexuality, even when it travels outside what mainstream culture deems acceptable. I haven't been able to feel the same sense of pride about my fatness – for me, the hatred and rejection is insidious and deeper and related to my inability to achieve certain goals (weight loss). Thinness is also the most highly prized measure my father used to establish success and acceptance. To feel happy to be fat is different to practicing daily acceptance of my fat body, and the fact that all but one of my sexual partners have appreciated and loved my fat body as it is, has shifted but not transformed my view of my fat body.

Is fat sex in front of a mirror taboo?

In 'Flaunting fat: sex with the lights on' (2014) I suggested that it is taboo in Western culture to be fat and naked and have sex with the lights on. Since then I have wondered if fat sex in front of a mirror is an even more taboo concept. My male partner Nick and I moved into a house a couple of weeks ago and it has floor-to-ceiling mirrored built-in-wardrobes in the master bedroom, a decorating decision I have always abhorred, and considered tacky. But, with a deep blue velvet bed frame, art deco dresser and chrome glass trolley, and bright throw rugs, there is a bohemian gothic opulence that could work with the floor-to-ceiling mirrors.

When I got out of bed one morning, my side facing the mirrors, I stared at my seated naked body. I found myself looking objectively, thinking, 'This is how my body looks now, four months after birthing my baby daughter'. My partner came into the room and said, 'How could you not love that body – just look at it!' I looked at it, and I thought, 'Whatever it is, it's already here'. It exists as it is; my shape has changed since before the pregnancy. My legs are slimmer, my back perhaps smoother, but my stomach is larger and heavier, and will droop more with time. I have realised the notion of 'getting your body back' after having a baby is a myth. You get it back, with permanent changes, especially when you're 37 as opposed to 23 years old. My breasts are full of milk, and will also droop when I stop breastfeeding. It is as it is.

But I looked back into the mirror and saw Nick's face reflected, admiration lighting it up, even more I think, since I carried and birthed and feed our baby with my fat body. I know he looks forward to seeing my body reflected in the mirror from different angles, as we have fat sex. I hope it will be soon, but moving house with a four month old, surrounded by boxes, demand feeding for hours a day, almost too exhausted to write this, we will see. We will keep the mirrored wardrobe for now and he will get the chance to explore his voyeuristic tendencies, and I may or may not angle myself to observe with interest.

References

Brophy, K. 1998, *Creativity: psychoanalysis, surrealism and creative writing*, University of Melbourne Press, Australia.

Going the Distance, 2010, New Line Cinema, USA. Directed by N. Burstein.

Kabat-Zinn, J. 2007, 'Three minute breathing space', Guided meditation practices CD in M. Williams, J. Teasdale, Z. Segal and J. Kabat-Zinn, *The mindful way through depression*, The Guilford Press, New York.

Lee, J. 2014, 'Flaunting fat: sex with the lights on', in S. Murray, C. Pause and J. Wykes (eds), *Queering Fat Embodiment*, Ashgate, Farnham.

Lee, J. 2013, 'My life as a superhero' in B. Olver (ed.), *Clones, fairies and monsters in the closet*, Big Pulp, USA.

Lee, J. 2007, 'Confessions of a female serial killer', *Verandah 22*, Deakin University, Australia.

McGregor, F. 1996, 'I am not a lesbian', in C. Berry and A. Jagose (eds), *Meanjin Literary Journal*, vol. 55, no. 1, pp. 31–46.

Pretty Woman, 1990, Touchstone Pictures, USA. Directed by G. Marshall.

When Harry Met Sally, 1989, Castle Rock Entertainment, USA. Directed by R. Reiner.

While You Were Sleeping, 1995, Hollywood Pictures, USA. Directed by J. Turteltaub.

The Pornography of Fat

Chapter 8
Queering Porn: Gender and Size Diversity within SF Bay Area Queer Pornography

Natalie Ingraham

Queer pornography is an emerging genre of pornography both in film and web-based explicit sexual content (Cork 2009). Pornography or porn is generally defined as a range of sexual representations designed to sexually excite consumers, although the definition of porn is also social: what is considered pornographic or sexually explicit varies in different historical, cultural and social contexts (Andrews 2012). This chapter explores queer pornography or "queer porn," a genre that includes lesbian, gay, bisexual, trans*[1], queer or genderqueer (LGBTQ) performers, or creators (including directors or producers). This definition is supported by participants who describe queer porn not based on the sexual acts featured but by the queer identity of the performers and producers creating the work. The academic study of porn has addressed issues of power, sexual expression, sexual health and a number of other topics related to human sexuality and health (Williams 2004a). Although other genres of porn have been addressed in academic writing, little to no attention has been given to fat bodies within pornography, including a lack of literature on BBW (Big Beautiful Women) pornography with a few notable exceptions (Goddard 2007; Flores 2014). This chapter focuses on the experiences of fat-identified performers and directors from within the queer porn community in the Bay Area of California. First, relevant literatures on the sexuality of fat bodies are reviewed followed by an introduction to the participants interviewed for this study and methods of analysis. The central theme of queer porn as community

1 The use of the term trans* reflects an adaption of web-based language taken up by the trans* community. The * (asterisk) is used as a wildcard in web searches by acting as a placeholder or a fill-in-the blank symbol. This symbol or representation has been applied to the gender identification to expand and include "folks who identify as transgender and transsexual (the terms usually understood as included when the prefix trans is used on its own) as well as other identities where a person does not identify with the gender they were assigned at birth" (Jones 2013).

is introduced to situate the rest of the main themes of the chapter. Analysis of queer porn debut narratives reveal activist leanings and motivations for pursuing queer porn work followed by a related discussion of the importance of visible fat, queer bodies on screen within queer porn and how these bodies are gendered. Finally, the implications of this study and future projects on the sexuality of fat bodies within pornography are discussed.

Asexual/Hypersexual Fat Bodies

Braziel and LeBesco's book, *Bodies Out of Bounds*, includes essays on fat sexuality that address both historical and modern views of fat sexuality through a variety of disciplinary lenses, from literary criticism to sociology to cultural studies (2001). Braziel writes that the fat body is often seen as diseased and deformed, while also undermining traditional philosophical binaries (dualisms) such as the gender binary in relationship to sexuality, especially for large women who are expected to be smaller and subordinated to men (2001, p.232). Braziel describes the fat body as an ambivalent body—at once asexual and hypersexual. Perspectives on the fat body vary according to audience and expectation. The asexual fat body derives from assumptions about a lack of sexual attractiveness with large body size while the hypersexual body reflects a connection between excess weight and excess pleasure, often-excessive food or drink. Braziel notes that fatness has also been associated with criminality and associated, in psychological literature, with destructive behaviour—a "body heedlessly embracing proscribed social mores" by its very existence (2001, p.3).

LeBesco (2004) discusses fat sexuality in her monograph by examining similarities between fat and queer embodied experiences. She contends that fatness is inherently queer by virtue of its "non-normative" existence. In addition, she finds that fat and queer communities share two things: the desire of some individuals (both within and outside the community) to find essential biological explanations for both states of being as well as the desire to find psychological pathologies as explanations for fatness and queerness, as both share the association with sexual deviance (LeBesco 2004, p.86). LeBesco also highlights specific variations within queer sexuality (e.g., gay male "bear" culture and butch lesbian body types).

Because it is a relatively new genre of porn, little critical scholarship focused specifically on queer porn and its surrounding community at the time of data collection, although more recent work addresses the growing complexity and need for critical porn studies (Attwood 2002; Attwood 2011; Ryberg 2012). Previous scholarly and journalistic essays attempted to define queer pornography (Cork 2009; Day 2009), but they did not necessarily pursue in-depth exploration with participants in this community to learn more about its shared meanings, values and identities, a gap in research that this study attempts to address. This chapter focuses specifically on the experiences of fat-identified individuals who participate in the production of queer pornography.

Study Design

This chapter analyses data from a mixed qualitative methods exploratory study of the queer pornography community in the San Francisco Bay Area of California. The project included in-depth interviews, participant observation and ethnographic field work with queer pornography producers, directors and performers. The purpose of the larger project was to explore queer pornography as one of many pornographies and highlight unique aspects of the genre, including the diversity of performers along various identities including race, gender and body size. The current chapter focuses mainly on the inclusion of fat bodies within queer pornography and how fat-identified performers within queer porn view their work as activism. Because queer porn is an understudied social world, triangulation of data via a combination of two qualitative methods is warranted. Ethnography was chosen because of its utility in observing and analysing previously unstudied or understudied groups (Emerson 2001). This is especially true vis-à-vis critical feminist ethnography where the body of the researcher plays a key role in the data collection (Bain and Nash 2006), as mine did during ethnographic observations of queer porn events. Although I did not participate in queer porn during my ethnographic data collection, my fat body was visible at all the queer porn events I attended as well as during the interview process. This visibility, in addition to my visible female/femme identity and my whiteness were all factors to consider during my analysis of the data. The methodology for this study is explored further in other work (see Ingraham 2013) but the two main data collection methods, narrative analysis and ethnography, are briefly discussed below.

Narrative Analysis

Narrative analysis focuses on oral or written stories told by participants to explore how they express "emotions, thoughts and interpretations" as well as how voices are constrained or enabled by other social forces (Chase 2005, p.656). Narratives can also do political work when utilized by groups of people to forge connections and foster social change (Plummer 1995). Specifically, how can the narrative of an individual be taken up by a group in the project of engaging in activism around visibility of identities? The process of exploring diverse identities as one aspect of narrative analysis drew me to consider it for this study, as I anticipated wide variation in how and why participants came to participate in queer porn. Interviewing was used to gather these narratives (Denzin and Lincoln 2005), with particular attention given to the interview itself as an interactive process (Enosh 2005).

Ethnographic Description

Ethnography involves in-depth observation and description of a culture or subculture that highlights the beliefs, practices and values of that social world in an empirically rich way (Emerson 2001). Ethnography was also an important methodological choice for this study because it connects directly to feminist methods through Dorothy Smith's work on standpoint theory[2] (1988). Other feminist methodologies also emphasize how individuals are "experts on the conditions of their own life" (Walby 2007, p.1011). The goal of ethnographic description highlighted here is to explore, briefly, how the connections among these individuals generate and sustain a community that produces queer porn.

Data Collection

Recruitment for this project was done entirely online, mainly through social networking websites (the BDSM/Kink site Fetlife, Facebook, and Twitter). The eight participants in this small study ranged in age from 19 to 30, and ranged in experience in porn from 1–10 years. Six of the eight were white, one identified as multi-racial and one identified as West Indian/African American; these participants are also referred to as People of Colour (POC) within this chapter. In terms of gender identity, I interviewed one cisgender male, three trans* men, two genderqueer people and two cisgender females.[3] All eight participants identified as queer and two of the four also identified as gay men in certain circles as well. Four of my eight participants identified at fat as well as being size positive or fat activists, both within and outside of their work in

2 Feminist standpoint theory (Smith 1988; Hartsock 1983) emphasizes the importance of recognizing your individual standpoint or perspective when taking on the study or observation of others as a way to strive for ethical and egalitarian principles as well as giving voice to the marginalized, especially in the context of qualitative research such as ethnography.

3 The National Center for Transgender Equality (2009) defines transgender as "an umbrella term for people whose gender identity, expression or behavior is different from those typically associated with their assigned sex at birth." The Gender Equity Resource Center (2013) at Berkeley defines genderqueer as "a person who redefines or plays with gender, or who refuses gender altogether." The website for Basic Rights Oregon, an LGBT rights organization, define cisgender (or cissexual) as a term that describes "people who, for the most part, identify as the gender they were assigned at birth" (Tash 2011).

queer porn. These four interviews are highlighted here in addition to more general themes from the data.

Main Themes: Community, Fat Visibility and Gender

Queer Porn as Community

This study began as a fusion of three research interests areas: fat studies, sexuality and media. Exploration and definition of queer porn as a community was the overarching goal with more specific probes to learn more about queer porn beliefs about sexuality, gender identity and body size. While all of the interviews mention the idea of a "queer porn community," experiences of this community differed for each person. Most participants mentioned using social networking websites to network among existing "friends" in the industry, as well as to seek out new contacts and shooting opportunities. For example, Facebook and Twitter were mentioned as venues where participants promote both themselves and their work, in addition to promoting queer porn social events, which are themselves closely connected to other common spaces found in the Bay Area LGBT/queer communities. James Darling, a white, trans man in his mid-twenties, described one particular queer porn social event and its connection to the Bay Area queer community:

> James: Um, it depends, you know. One example is when I went to help [Courtney Trouble] with her Queer Porn TV fundraiser party thing. There was a ton of queer people there. And it was awesome to see us like all at the same places and certain kinds of events and because we're queers. You know, the queer community is small to begin with, so at different queer dance parties or different events, you're probably going to see queer porn stars um, hanging out because that's just the nature of being in that just even smaller—tiny bubble.

A few participants commented on the use of common spaces and sharing spaces with the LGBTQ community more broadly (Anderson et al. 2010). In fact, three of the four queer porn events I attended as part of my fieldwork were held at LGBTQ venues. Two were at the same queer bar in the Mission District[4] and another at a distinctly lesbian bar nearby. Below are excerpts from my field notes describing one such space:

---

4 The Mission District is San Francisco's oldest neighborhood and was historically a working-class neighborhood with mainly Spanish-speaking (Latino/Chicano) immigrant populations. In recent years, the neighborhood as seen a demographic shift/gentrification to a younger, whiter population. The Mission has a number of queer/

> The second launch party for QueerPorn.TV was at the Lexington Club, a small lesbian/queer bar in the Mission District of San Francisco. "The Lex" is quite small, very much a "dive" bar with two tiny bathroom stalls, labelled without gender assignment. Local art lines the dark painted walls. Walking in on this night was overwhelming. Music was blasting from the corner DJ booth, little more than a card table with some laptops and speakers. The bar was jammed with at least 75 people in various postures—standing, crowded around the tiny tables, across the wall from the bar, or elbowing in at the bar to get a drink from the bartenders. A television set played clips from the various shoots for the pay portion of QueerPorn.TV. This meant that discussions about my friend's day at work were interspersed with quick glimpses of naked bodies, whips, gloves and even the occasional sex sling—none of which really fazed me for the most part.

Here we see the blurred boundaries that exemplify the hybridities of the queer porn community and larger LGBT communities of the San Francisco Bay Area. This fieldwork and the commentaries of the participants themselves strongly support the idea of a queer porn community, as fluid in nature as the word queer itself.

Defining Queer Porn

Many definitions of the queer porn community provided by participants reflect the challenges of defining a porn genre. This struggle to define queer porn was often ameliorated by using a comparative method of definition rather than definitive statements about queer meanings per se. That is, participants largely described it more broadly in terms of what it is *not*—things and people it does not include in its existence as a queer entity. Queer porn, much like the theoretical notion of queering a concept, exists for these participants as a shift in the way porn is conceptualized, produced, and consumed. This was most often clarified through explicit comparisons with "mainstream" porn, both straight (female/male) and gay (male/male). Courtney Trouble, a fat-identified, white, genderqueer[5] porn producer and actor, started their first queer porn company, No Fauxxx, in 2004 and currently runs Indie Porn Revolution and Queerporn.tv. Here, Courtney describes how No Fauxxx began when they noticed a lack of bodies and relationships like theirs in existing alternative porn.

LGBT bars including El Rio, The Lex(ington), and a few Latin@ LGBT bars as well, reflecting its neighborhood reputation for nightlife.

5 At the time of the interview for this study, Courtney Trouble identified as female. However, Courtney came out in 2013 as genderqueer, thus they/them pronouns are used to describe them in this chapter (C. Trouble 2013, personal communcation, 29 October).

Courtney Trouble: Queer porn, like the term queer porn did not exist up until about 6 year ago [2004] and I started No Fauxxx almost 10 years ago, so. But back then it was being called alt porn … There was stuff being made that I would, in retrospect, call queer porn. But nobody really called it that. One of No Fauxxx's mottos was "subversive smut made by ladies, artists and queers." That was its motto and then the queer thing started to pick up and I said fuck it … .Yeah, I think queer is such a- could be- just has diversity written into it as far as the queer, GLBT movement- has such a diverse stamp on it already that is perfect for porn that describes you know a group of people who live outside of these clichéd realms.

Sophia St. James, a fat-identified, cisgender female, Black/West Indian actor, commented on the nature of queer porn and its growing popularity, noting concern about queer porn losing some of its activist or radical roots to larger, mainstream porn forces. Sophia also importantly notes the lack of "sizeism" in queer porn and how it embraces diverse body types, including larger bodies like her own. While she felt that queer porn currently avoids the pitfalls of "niche" genres such as BBW or ethnicity-based porn, she shares a concern that mainstream porn might try to appropriate queer porn in the same way.

Sophia St. James: Right. I see queer porn- I see people within mainstream porn turning queer porn into a niche. I see that mainstream porn taking queer porn and saying, "Oh, this is just like gay porn, BBW porn, Black porn, Asian porn" and making it- be the next fetish—queer porn. And it will become commercialized. If or unless those of us within queer porn prevent that. Of course, like I would love to see queer porn get nominations and awards from the big, top people but not if that means selling your soul. And, I would love to see queer porn make a name for itself and say, "Here we are. We exist." But it doesn't mean that I want to join in the rat race of the mainstream porn world. It would be really cool to see it recognized without having to become a niche. I feel niches are another way of being racist, homophobic, [or] sexist. [laughs] Anyway, that's my hope—that it doesn't get to that point.

N. Ingraham: And for right now, for you, it doesn't feel like queer porn is those things?

Sophia: Oh, absolutely not. I feel queer porn is not- is like, absolutely not racist, obviously not homophobic [laughs]. There's no like sizeism, there's no- sexiness and sex appeal comes in a variety of packages, looks, shapes, sizes and because of that, we want- or queer porn showcases that so that way it appeals to all queers or all individuals who enjoy queer porn.

Although Sophia doesn't make the connection directly, parallels exist between BBW porn and queer porn in terms of the way both challenge heteronormative ideas of sexiness in porn. In his piece on BBW porn, Goddard argues that "BBW is not merely a variant of normative sexuality but a range of practices that potentially submit the foundation of heterosexual normativity to a profound questioning from within" going on to say that BBW might even be set up as a "sexual identity, along the lines of gay, lesbian and trans sexual identities" (2007, p.193). Stealth Machine, one of the fat-identified genderqueer performers, described queer porn as a showcase for a variety of "non-normalized" sexualities and clearly distinguished between queer porn and mainstream porn by its intended audience.

> Stealth Machine: I think queer porn is porn that showcases non-normalized sexualities and genders. And I think defining queer as non-normalized behaviour kind of sums up queer porn. It's non-normalized porn. So you can have two women fucking on screen, but if those two women aren't actually queer or bi or gay identified, and are doing it for a male gaze, then it's not queer because that's the normalized form of pornography for a cisgender male audience. Versus two women fucking on screen who are both queer or bi or gay identified and are doing it for other women, I think is non-normalized in the porn industry ... I think kinky porn to a certain extent is queer porn because it's non-normalized sexual behaviour that's happening on screen. Trans* people fucking on screen in a way that's not fetishized is non-normalized in the porn industry. Trans men fucking on screen is queer porn because it's not really seen in the [mainstream] porn industry.

Here, we also see that queer porn was described as distinct from gay, lesbian or heterosexual porn because of performers' various gender presentations, especially non-binary genders (trans* or genderqueer) rarely featured in other types of porn.

Narratives of Debut and Visible Fat Bodies

Participants' debut stories, accounts of how they got started in queer porn, were quite diverse. Many participants had gotten into the business through a sexual partner (most participants use the term "lover" since almost all of the people I interviewed are in open or polyamorous relationships). Below is one condensed version of Sophia's debut in queer porn.

> Sophia St. James: [laughs] Okay. So, I fell one day, ripped my meniscus and broke my elbow and I was laid up in bed, couldn't do anything and was Googling.

> I ... ended up coming across an article about how Madison Young brought Syd Blackovich to an award [show] ... So, of course I Googled Syd Blackovich and then I saw Pink & White and Crashpad and all these things pop up. And this was 2 years and—yeah about two years [ago] and I've been an off and on sex worker since I was 19. So, the idea of me doing porn wasn't too farfetched but it just never was something that- I never really thought about it because I didn't fit the typical porn look. Um, but I saw [Syd] and I started becoming obsessed with it. Like, San Francisco's not that far away, I would love to do something with this. So after talking with my partner, I ended up filling out a [model] application [for a queer porn website].

Although Sophia was engaged with other forms of sex work before starting in queer porn, she, like other participants (both fat and not-fat), expressed a desire to do queer porn specifically because of the freedom it offered in terms of identity expression. It allowed Sophia to make her queer, female, larger body of colour more visible in a genre of porn that would value her as an intersectional individual rather than "assigning" her to marked space in BBW (Big Beautiful Women) or "ethnic" (read: minority) porn. She described these as "typical niche porn" such as "ebony porn," saying, "I didn't want to categorize myself like that and the only way that you could do mainstream porn is if you choose to do that."

Black feminist scholar Miller-Young asserts that pornography is a "racialized economy of desire" (2008, p. 229) or what Kipnis (1999, p.164) calls a "racialized political theater" with the creation of black and interracial porn as sub-genres of mainstream pornography only in the last 20 years. Linda Williams (2004b) also discusses race in porn via an analysis of interracial porn, though her work focused on specific heterosexual examples rather than queer porn specifically. Other studies of gay male pornography find support for racist imagery of Black and Latino actors (Hernandez and Tester 2004). Although none of my participants expressed concern about racist images of people of colour in queer porn, Sophia even calling queer porn "not racist" specifically, a common complaint among both participants of colour and white participants concerned the "whiteness" of most queer porn, a fact reflected in the racial/ethnic makeup of my participants as well. Lance Armstar, a trans man of colour, told me about his first queer porn experience that made visible not just his trans body but also his body of colour. Lance saw a casting call asking specifically for lesbian women of colour to do an all POC [People of Colour] porn shoot. He thought to himself, "'Hell yeah!' And then I showed up and I was like, 'I don't really identify as a woman, what do you guys think about this?' So that was really neat." Lance found this queer porn shoot not just accepting his trans male body but celebrating it in order to explicitly feature queer people of colour.

Stealth Machine echoed other debut stories from trans and genderqueer performers who wanted to make such bodies more visible on screen. However, Stealth Machine was unique in transitioning into on screen work not through a lover but rather through doing behind the scenes work on other queer porn projects as a photographer and videographer.

> Stealth Machine: I was scared I think because I have such a boner for [their co-star]. So it was anxiety around that. And also because it was my first time fucking on screen. I guess I didn't mention that I had done a couple of the Public Disgraces with Kink.com. So I had been on screen before in a porn shoot, but clothed. I hadn't been the one getting fucked. It was always me pulling a cock out of my pants and having someone suck it. It's more anonymous when your clothes are on. I also was really grateful that I expressed to [costar] that I had a lot of concerns about how much of my body that I wanted to show. I'm not dysphoric for gender reasons, its more, even though I'm a proud fat person and whatever, I think there's still a shame and fear around showing my belly or whatever. And how that's going to … I think there's that fear of bullying that comes up. And [costar] was really supportive. She's like, "You can leave all your clothes on or take them all off. I don't care." In the end, because I'm a big slut, I took all my clothes off. Which I'm really happy I did. For political reasons, I think it was really important for me to get naked on camera.

Courtney Trouble's debut also reflected a desire to see "bodies like mine" on screen when they started their first queer porn company over ten years ago. Today they continue to work to make their porn more inclusive not only of people of colour but also of trans/genderqueer bodies, fat bodies and bodies at intersections of all of these identities.

> *N. Ingraham*: What other things were missing for you in mainstream porn that you wanted to showcase?
>
> *Courtney Trouble*: I mean, it was purely selfish. I didn't see any like fat, tattooed nerdy girls, you know. [laughs] In these big budget pictures, not that I would ever expect that to change now, although April Flores [a BBW performer] but-yeah, so I didn't see. It's not like I wanted to jerk off to girls that looked like me, it was more, wanting to fit in more than being aroused or wanting to watch porn with me in it. It was more the principle of it. Um, and mainstream porn is never going to do that but indie porn and DIY porn- it's so easy to make porn. Anybody can do it. All you need is a camera so the whole idea of indie or DIY porn, of being able to represent yourself be it size or gender or race or sexuality. It's possible for anybody … . Like, I didn't really- as far as diversity goes, I didn't really set out trying to have this many trans men, this many plus size [sic], like

> trying to make it an equal playing around. I never set out with that pie shaped diversity plan, I just wanted everything to feel open and so now you know when the numbers are way, way up and you know, I'm working with so many different kinds of people and doing all these different projects and performing myself.

Stealth Machine was also quite explicit in describing their activism-based reasons for deciding to do queer porn:

> Stealth Machine: I think adding onto that, though, I think it's non-normalized but it's also porn with intention. Most queer porn does it with radical politics attached. So they're thinking about the health and well being of the models, and thinking about that gaze and all that academic shit. I think that also sets it apart. This isn't just fucking on screen, this is fucking on screen because we want to, as Madison Young said, record our sexuality. Or because we don't see our bodies on screen.

Despite their quite different debuts into queer porn (e.g., through a lover, through an online modelling application), the participants shared a common motivation of increasing visibility of their bodies and, moreover, had positive experiences that led them to continue doing queer porn. To them, this type of work is more than just a source of income, but rather a form of activism that uses the visibility of their bodies and their sexuality to queer ideas of what porn can and should look like. Stealth Machine, like others, directly identified their reason for moving from behind the scenes to onscreen work in queer porn was for "political reasons," a passionate desire to use their fat, genderqueer body to advocate for the expansion of what is considered sexy by recording their sexuality and their fat body for consumption by queer porn viewers. Courtney Trouble echoed this, noting their first website was designed to showcase "fat, nerdy" bodies and personalities like their own and those of their friends; a direct action to represent their non-normative fat and queer bodies otherwise ignored by the mainstream porn industry.

Gender and Fatness Within Queer Porn

Much of the writing on fatness and sexuality focuses on women's fat bodies specifically. Cecilia Hartley approaches the topic of fat sexuality via feminist scholarship in her essay in Braziel and LeBesco's *Body Out of Bounds* (2001). She echoes Braziel's assertion that fat body exists in a state of simultaneous lack and excess of sexuality. Fat storage on women's bodies tends to be in areas considered "sexy" (e.g., breasts, hips and derriere) but this body is also often considered asexual. LeBesco (2004) addresses fat sexuality by noting similarities between fat and queer embodied experiences. She contends that fatness is inherently queer by virtue of its "non-normative" existence. In addition, she finds that fat and queer communities share two things: the desire of some individuals (both within and outside the community) to find essential biological explanations for both states of being, as well as the desire to find psychological pathologies as explanations for both states. LeBesco also writes on specific variations within queer sexuality around body size e.g., gay male "bear" culture that privileges and eroticizes large, hairy male bodies (Hennen 2008) and butch lesbian body types. LeBesco notes that "though there's plenty of disdain for fat in queer circles" she retains interest in the possibility for fat positive activism in the queer community, noting that "supportive queer communities nurture their members, whatever size or shape, recognizing 'that to be cruel' (90); dismissive, or judgmental of each other plays into the hands of those who actively promote antigay agenda" (19). Participants in this study discussed the inclusively wide range of gender presentations as one accolade for queer porn, listing it among the diversity showcased in queer porn productions. However, fat-identified performers, both genderqueer and male, held a more nuanced view of how fatness is presented in queer porn.

Stealth Machine described their reasons for transitioning from behind the camera to being in front of the camera for their first on-screen performance in queer porn as being directly related to the lack of fat genderqueer visibility in queer porn.

> Stealth Machine: I see a lot of fat femmes in porn, and how fat feminine bodies seem to be more normalized in both mainstream and in queer porn. And I don't see a lot of fat trans male or female-bodied transmasculine[6] whatever folks. I don't see a lot of fat trans women, either. And that was really frustrating to me. And although I was totally wrapped up in this queer porn revolution and really excited about it, I wasn't seeing my body on screen. Which was frustrating, and one of the biggest motivating reasons I decided to porn. Because I was like, "I don't want to bitch about it, I want to do something about it." So, in making the decision to actually take my [chest] binder off, was not wanting to hide.

Stealth Machine emphasized that most of the larger bodies in queer porn are those of fat femmes, or feminine queer women and that the bodies of small/thin trans men are often eroticized, which they felt reflected the larger queer community and its reluctance to embrace fat sexuality. The participants

6 Transmasculine is a term that refers to transgender individuals who tend to be more masculine than feminine. As (Saltzburg 2010) notes that although "FTM transsexual" is an identity that many on the transmasculine spectrum claim it is one which does not fit everyone with a transmasculine identity.

who talked about their body size most explicitly were also fat-identified. For them, much like the trans/genderqueer participants, being in queer porn was a way to make their bodies visible on screen. Not only are their bodies made more visible, but also the spectrum of fat sexuality is made more visible—no small feat considering the fat shaming rhetoric that includes assumptions of asexuality among fat folks noted by LeBesco and others such as Murray (2004) and Gailey (2012).

My first two interviews were with two gay and queer identified men who were also partners, Ian Sparks and Brett McCloskey. Both men are also fat-identified, although neither mentioned engaging in a lot of fat-specific activism. Ian runs two different queer porn production companies; one focused on queer men, both cisgender and transgender, called T-Wood [formerly TrannyWood] and a more gender diverse company called Dolores Park Studios. Brett has only been involved in a few productions of Ian's from T-Wood. Both men described T-Wood's intentional inclusion of larger bodies, mainly to reflect the diversity within the gay "bear" culture.

> *Ian Sparks*: Our quandary at the beginning was- well, the two ideas were- we could do real bears of colour because normally in bear films you see mainly white guys and maybe one black guy, maybe in another film you'll see some Latin[o] guys. Um, and we just knew from our friends and our customers that, okay, that's not reality.

> *Brett McCloskey*: Uh, you know, and as far as body types, yeah, we definitely ran the gamut from, you know, very thin and muscular to much more you know, round and bearish and furry like myself. And so yeah, that was a fun thing to see how different body types worked together and worked together on film. And you learn certain angles do and do not work when you put two larger fellows together versus a larger person and a slightly smaller or mid built actors. So sometimes there's a learning curve [laughs] there. You're like, well that looked great on paper but the physics are a little different and again, just our great ability to just kind of go, "Okay, we've got to improvise here and change this up a little bit and make it work." Yeah, that's and also the diversity in experiences too … So, um, yeah, and even diversity in tattoos, piercings, some guys didn't have ink, some guys had a lot of ink. And a little bit of everything. Again, that's part of the joy.

Brett was the only participant to really comment on the "nitty gritty" details of how porn production or sexual activity changes when fat bodies are included, such as the need to think differently about sex positions or lighting issues. Generally, the main reason many participate in queer porn (as opposed to other types of sex work) is their ability to "tell stories" to consumers with their bodies in ways not allowed in mainstream porn due to gender or race or body shape, either through exclusion from mainstream porn altogether or ghettoization into fetish porn. This seemed especially true for the fat-identified participants who sought to make their fat sexuality visible in this specific way via queer porn participation.

Discussion

Building on previous research of queer porn (Day 2009; Hernandez and Tester 2004), this study adds to the literature through an empirical exploration of a queer pornography community and its fat-identified members. This study provides a foundation for further research on this community to its embodied activism. Labelling this group as a community also holds promise for addressing the topic of pornography via a number of sociological avenues including the sociology of work in porn, the sociology of emotions in partner negotiations, and the sociology of sexuality including sexual identity, meanings of sex acts, etc. This unique blending of activism and work attempts and often succeeds in making queer and fat sexuality visible in a commoditized product available to the queer community and beyond. Research on queer porn by Lipton (2012) since data collection for this project supports the activism and body diversity highlighted here.

One question raised during the process of this study and subsequent presentations and discussions is the question of fatness as "queer." This definition asks for a broadening of sociological understandings of "queer" beyond the realm of sexualities and genders to include other forms of embodiment that resist normative social imperatives. I don't think of fat as inherently queer as it feels important to keep queer as a term and signifier for gender and sexuality. I think fatness can and does certainly resist normative social imperatives about bodies, as in the case of the two genderqueer participants or even my two trans participants. Discussing fatness as queer presents an interesting intellectual exercise, but I would find it problematic if a fat-identified person identified as queer solely because of their body size. It is important to make and hold space for queer identities formed via non-heteronormative genders and sexualities and I worry that adding in fat as queer would allow privileged cisgender or heterosexual fat-identified individuals to encroach or appropriate the word.

However, I also agree with writers like Anna Mollow (2013a; 2013b), who argues that queer movements can and must include fat liberation in their social justice pursuits. I think fatness is certainly part of intersectional identities that contribute to our personal and social understandings of gender and sexuality. For Stealth Machine and Sophia, their fatness is something that certainly relates to both aspects of their identities. For Sophia, it was about connecting her race, size and sexuality in a way that went beyond niche pornography and fetishism. She found that queer porn was the porn "home" of sorts that could showcase the many facets of who she was as a person without categorizing her into a BBW or what she considered offensive porn based on her race. For Stealth Machine, race wasn't as explicit in their narrative, perhaps because they are white, so their fatness and gender identity were the most salient aspects of identity in the context of their work in queer porn. However, I don't think either of them thought of their body size, their "non-normative bodies" as queer because of their size alone—it was more about their gender and/or sexuality that identified them as such. Courtney Trouble also identified as a fat woman at the time of the interview, but I didn't find anything in their narrative that pointed to feeling that her fat body their queer on its own.

A colleague also asked about the possibility of building solidarity across social movements if fat was considered queer. I think that there is still this possibility and actually, within the fat acceptance or size acceptance community, a real need to open up to other communities especially around gender fluidity and race. The fat acceptance movement historically and today is largely, white, female and cisgender (in my experience). Although there has certainly been a historical connection between fat activism and lesbian or queer activism (Hill 2009; Saguy 2013), most agree that fat activism could benefit from intersectional approaches to visible bodies described by my participants. In fact, this has been an increasingly central topic in more radical fat spaces such as the annual NOLOSE conference, described as a "vibrant community of fat queers and our allies, with a shared commitment to feminist, anti-oppression ideology and action, seeking to end the oppression of fat people" (NOLOSE 2010). Listening and learning from fat queer individuals or fat trans individuals or fat POC (or fat POC trans/queer folks, etc.) about their experiences can only serve to strengthen the community.

While queer porn has certainly tried to be as inclusive as possible, there is also a fair and common criticism that queer porn doesn't always try hard enough to move outside the thin ideal in its representations of queer bodies—or for that matter, bodies of colour and bodies of trans women in particular (Steinbock 2014). While body size has been considered in our understandings of gender and sexuality for some time, fatness itself as the focal point for gender and sexuality critique is a newer phenomenon in academia. I think it makes more sense to think about fatness, queer sexuality and trans and genderqueer bodies as being transgressive or boundary blurring if not boundary breaking in similar but distinct ways.

Acknowledgements

I would like to thank Dr. Adele Clarke for her guidance during the research and writing process. Dr. Shari Dworkin for editing assistance and Dr. Carla A. Pfeffer for her thoughtful feedback on this content during conference proceedings. I would also like to thank Caroline Walters and Helen Hester for their helpful edits to this chapter.

References

Anderson, J., Adey, P. and Bevan, P., 2010. Positioning place: polylogic approaches to research methodology. *Qualitative Research*, 10(5), pp.589–604.

Andrews, D., 2012. Toward A More Valid Definition of "Pornography." *The Journal of Popular Culture*, 45(3), pp.457–477.

Attwood, F., 2002. Reading Porn: The Paradigm Shift in Pornography Research. *Sexualities*, 5(1), pp.91–105.

Attwood, F., 2011. The Paradigm Shift: Pornography Research, Sexualisation and Extreme Images: The Paradigm Shift. *Sociology Compass*, 5(1), pp.13–22.

Bain, A.L. and Nash, C.J., 2006. Undressing the researcher: feminism, embodiment and sexuality at a queer bathhouse event. *Area*, 38(1), pp.99–106.

Braziel, J.E. and LeBesco, K., 2001. *Bodies Out of Bounds: Fatness and Transgression*, Berkeley: University of California Press.

Chase, S., 2005. Narrative Inquiry: Multiple Lenses, Approaches, Voices. In *Handbook of Qualitative Research*, Thousand Oaks, CA: Sage.

Cork, A., 2009. The Queer Porn Revolution | The Skinny. Available at: http://www.theskinny.co.uk/deviance/features/45067-the_queer_porn_revolution [Accessed September 16, 2012].

Day, A., 2009. *Feminism and Pornography after the Sex Wars: Diversifying Pornography*, Los Angeles, CA: UC Los Angeles: UCLA Center for the Study of Women. Available at: http://www.escholarship.com/uc/item/61k265vv.

Denzin, N.K. and Lincoln, Y.S., 2005. *The Sage Handbook of Qualitative Research*, Thousand Oaks, Calif.: Sage Publications.

Emerson, R.M., 2001. The Face of Contemporary Ethnography. In *Contemporary Field Research: Perspectives and Formulations*. Prospect Heights, IL: Waveland Press, pp. 27–53.

Enosh, G., 2005. The Interactive Construction of Narrative Styles in Sensitive Interviews: The Case of Domestic Violence Research. *Qualitative Inquiry*, 11(4), pp.588–617.

Flores, April. 2013. "Being Fatty D: Size, Beauty, and Embodiment in the Adult Industry." In *Feminist Porn Book*, 279–83. New York, N.Y.: the Feminist Press at CUNY.

Gailey, J.A., 2012. Fat Shame to Fat Pride: Fat Women's Sexual and Dating Experiences. *Fat Studies*, 1(1), pp.114–127.

Gender Equity Resource Center, 2013. Definition of Terms | UC Berkeley Gender Equity Resource Center. Available at: http://geneq.berkeley.edu/lgbt_resources_definiton_of_terms#gender_queer [Accessed January 18, 2013].

Goddard, M., 2007. BBW: Techno-Archaism, Excessive Corporeality and Network Sexuality. In K. Jacobs, M. Janssen, and M. Pasquinelli, eds. *CLICKME: A Netporn Studies Reader*. Amsterdam: Institute of Network Cultures, pp. 187–195.

Hartsock, N.C.M., 1983. The Feminist Standpoint: Developing the Ground For A Specifically Feminist Historical Materialism. In S. Harding and M. B. Hintikka, eds. *Discovering Reality*. D. Reidel Publishing Company, pp. 283–310.

Hennen, P., 2008. *Faeries, Bears, and Leathermen: Men in Community Queering the Masculine*, Chicago: University of Chicago Press.

Hernandez, M. and Tester, G., 2004. A Work in Progress: Doing Gender and Race in Queer Pornography. In *ASA Graduate Student Research-in-Progress Roundtable Session*. American Sociological Association Annual Meeting.

Hill, A.C., 2009. *Spatial Awarishness: Queer Women and the Politics of Fat Embodiment*. Thesis. Bowling Green State University.

Ingraham, N., 2013. Queering Pornography Through Qualitative Methods. *International Journal of Multiple Research Approaches*, pp.3969–3992.

Jones, Nash. 2013. "Bridging The Gap - Trans*: What Does the Asterisk Mean and Why Is It Used? | Q Center." *The Q Center*. August 8. http://www.pdxqcenter.org/bridging-the-gap-trans-what-does-the-asterisk-mean-and-why-is-it-used/.

Kipnis, L., 1999. *Bound and Gagged: Pornography and the Politics of Fantasy in America*, Durham, N.C.: Duke University Press.

LeBesco, K., 2004. *Revolting bodies?: The Struggle to Redefine Fat Identity*, Amherst, MA: University of Massachusetts Press.

Lipton, Shawna. 2012. "Trouble Ahead: Pleasure, Possibility and the Future of Queer Porn." *New Cinemas: Journal of Contemporary Film* 10 (2): 197–207. doi:10.1386/ncin.10.2-3.197_1.

Miller-Young, M., 2008. Hip-Hop Honeys and Da Hustlaz: Black Sexualities in the New Hip-Hop Pornography. *Represetin': Women, Hip-Hop, and Popular Music*, 8(1), pp.261–292.

Mollow, A., 2013a. Fat Liberation is Totally Queer | Bitch Media. *Bitch Media*. Available at: http://bitchmagazine.org/post/fat-liberation-is-totally-queer [Accessed October 31, 2013].

Mollow, A., 2013b. Sized Up | Bitch Media. *Bitch Media*. Available at: http://bitchmagazine.org/article/sized-up-fat-feminist-queer-disability [Accessed October 31, 2013].

Murray, S., 2004. Locating Aesthetics: Sexing the Fat Woman. *Social Semiotics*, 14(3), pp.237–247.

National Center for Transgender Equality, 2009. *Transgender Terminology*, Washington, DC: National Center for Transgender Equality.

NOLOSE, 2010. *nolose: the revolution just got bigger*. Available at: http://www.nolose.org/ [Accessed June 1, 2013].

Plummer, K., 1995. *Telling Sexual Stories: Power, Change, and Social Worlds*, London: New York: Routledge.

Ryberg, I., 2012. *Imagining Safe Space: The Politics of Queer, Feminist and Lesbian Pornography*, Stockholm: Acta Universitatis Stockholmiensis.

Saguy, A.C., 2013. *What's Wrong with Fat?*, New York: Oxford University Press.

Saltzburg, N.L., 2010. *Developing a Model of Transmasculine Identity*. Dissertation. Coral Gables, Florida: University of Miami.

Smith, D.E., 1988. *The Everyday World as Problematic: A Feminist Sociology*, Milton Keynes, England; New York: Open University Press.

Steinbock, E. 2014. "Pornography." *TSQ: Transgender Studies Quarterly* 1 (1-2): 156–58. doi:10.1215/23289252-2399893.

Tash, 2011. Trans 101: Cisgender: Basic Rights Oregon. Available at: http://www.basicrights.org/uncategorized/trans-101-cisgender/ [Accessed February 18, 2013].

Walby, K., 2007. On the Social Relations of Research: A Critical Assessment of Institutional Ethnography. *Qualitative Inquiry*, 13(7), pp.1008–1030.

Williams, L., 2004a. *Porn Studies*, Durham: Duke University Press.

Williams, L., 2004b. Pornography, Race, and Class: Skin Flicks on the Racial Border: Pornography, Exploitation, and Interracial Lust. In *Porn Studies*. Duke University Press, pp. 271–208.

Chapter 9

Bodies Like Our Own? The Dynamics of Distance and Closeness in Online Fat Porn

Goda Klumbyte and Katrine Smiet

Introduction

In 2009 the major adult industry magazine *Adult Video News* released its first issue with a BBW (Big Beautiful Women) model on the cover and a feature article about the BBW porn industry—a signal that pornography featuring fat female bodies is no longer an anomaly, but has reached a mainstream position in the adult entertainment landscape. However, like pornography in general, fat porn also has raised discussions about its potential merits and harms to "real life" fat women. Questions about whether BBW/fat pornography empowers fat women to claim and express their sexualities, or whether it objectifies them and perpetuates stereotypes are still as acute now as they were in 1979 when Carole Shaw coined the term BBW for her magazine.[1]

Fat women themselves often have a quite ambiguous relation to BBW/fat porn: while some claim that porn featuring fat bodies can help them to "get closer" to their bodies, others feel the distance growing larger due to the fetishization of the fat body in porn. In this chapter, we analyse the dynamic of distance and closeness between the fat body image in pornography and fat embodied subjectivities. Specifically, with porn production and consumption going online, we will investigate the role of the medium in this dynamic, and what kind of spaces of potentiality for fat women's sexual subjectivities are opened up by network technology. We use the term "fat porn" to encompass all kinds of pornographies that feature fat bodies, and we refer to "BBW porn" to talk about specific category of "Big Beautiful Women" porn. The main difference, as we see it, is that BBW porn focuses on specific expression of gender, which is the image of a highly feminine heterosexual woman, whereas

1 See: "BBW Magazine: Past and Present," http://bbwmagazine.com/pastandpresent_3.htm (accessed on December 6, 2013).

fat porn, in our view, is more of an "umbrella-term" that incorporates both BBW genre, but also, for instance, porn that features queer fat bodies.

Bringing together porn studies, phenomenological and new media approaches, the chapter will draw examples from BBW porn websites and will analyse responses to BBW/fat porn in a pro-fat web-forum. Exploring the multi-layered entanglement of the fat body and the imagery of fat porn, we argue that there is no clear either/or answer to the question of women's empowerment through fat pornography. Rather, it is an experience of resonance (Paasonen 2011) that characterizes the relation between embodied fat sexual subjects and pornography. By effectively enacting both processes of distancing and bringing closer at the same time, this body-image resonance opens up spaces of potential as well as constraint in lived experience of fatness.

Approaching Bodies and Experiences Through Phenomenology

In this chapter, we approach the body from a *feminist phenomenological* perspective. Feminist phenomenology combines classical phenomenological insights with an attention to how gendered structures are embodied and incorporated in lived experience. In this section, we shortly introduce the feminist phenomenological perspective, and the tools that it provides us to study weighing and desiring embodied selves.

In contrast to a long tradition of mind/body dualism in Western philosophical thinking, the phenomenological perspective considers mind and body as fundamentally intertwined. Phenomenology understand the body not just as a "thing in the world," but rather as a mediator of world: as our means of interacting *in* the world. Philosopher Edmund Husserl first made a clear distinction between the body as object and as a living being. The objectified body is the body as approached by science and medicine: it is primarily considered as a very complex biological organism, a "thing" which we can heal when it is sick, fix when it is broken (Welton 1998). The lived body on the other hand, is a body as it is lived and experienced by the subject. It refers to the body as a subject that perceives, as a body that is dynamic and active (ibid.). As Maurice Merleau-Ponty expressed it: "The body is the vehicle of being in the world" (1945/2002: 94). In other words, instead of thinking of human beings as disembodied minds, phenomenological perspective stresses that embodiment is central to our being.

Although classical phenomenologists such as Husserl, Heidegger and Merleau-Ponty have pioneered this embodied and non-dualist perspective on bodies and selves, we are indebted to feminist phenomenologists and queer phemenonologists such as Iris Marion Young and Sara Ahmed for the way in which they have made phenomenology relevant to contemporary concerns. A central achievement of feminist phenomenology of the body lies in making classical phenomenology sensitive to *difference*, notably the differences that exist in embodied experiences. Instead of taking the male, white and able-bodied body as an unacknowledged starting point for a supposedly neutral and universal description of the structures of human being-in-the-world, feminist phenomenology stresses that "the body" as such does not exist. Corporeality and lived experience, feminist phenomenologists contend, are fundamentally affected by embodied differences such as gender and race.

In other words, the phenomenological focus on the "lived body" and "lived experience" should not exclude or preclude attention to the level of societal structures. As feminist phenomenologist Iris Marion Young has pointed out, structures of inequality are not separate from embodied experiences but instead fundamentally shape them (2005). As a result, the study of lived experience can bring to light underlying norms and rules that govern those experiences. Relating this to the question of lived experiences of the weighing body, we can note that the dominant societal ideas around weight significantly shape individual experiences of fatness or thinness. The fat body, just as the thin body, does not exist in a cultural vacuum, but is lived in a society that attaches certain values and meanings to this body. To live the fat body in a contemporary Western society is to inhabit a body that is generally seen as unhealthy, unattractive and unwelcome (Lebesco 2004, Murray 2008b, Tischner 2012). Not surprisingly, the societal contempt for fat bodies has an influence on how the fat-bodied person experiences their own embodied self.

By recognizing how cultural norms and structures affect lived embodied experiences, feminist phemenologists have called into question the classical phenomenological distinction between "body image" and "body schema." Body image refers to a third-person perspective on the body: the body as it is seen by others. Body schema, on the other hand, is understood as referring to a pre-reflective first-person embodied experience: that is to say, how I experience my body "from the inside." However, this neat distinction between body image and body schema disintegrates in a context where the third-person perspective becomes integral to the first-person embodied self. The "attitude of others" is thus not external to lived experience, but instead societal imaginaries are literally incorporated and influence how one acts and engages in the world (for instance, see Iris Marion Young 2005).

What is "Fat"? On Fat Studies and Fat Acceptance

Because it stresses the importance of different intersections of structural categories in shaping embodied experiences, feminist phenomenology is a relevant tool for Fat Studies and the Fat Acceptance movement. In this chapter, our use of the word "fat" to describe a genre of pornography and a type of body is in line with the way the word has been reclaimed by Fat Studies scholars and Fat Acceptance activists. "Fat," as Samantha Murray has shown, is not a neutral word (2008a). She makes clear that on the basis of the visible appearance of the body, conclusions are easily made about eating habits (food addict) and life styles (inactive)—but also about character traits (lazy, defiant) and values (moral failure, out of control). Indeed, fatness is culturally framed as a health transgression, an aesthetic transgression, and consequently often even as a moral transgression. Analyzing and challenging this negative cultural construction of fatness, Fat Studies scholars have opened up spaces for more positive understandings of fat. The emergent and blossoming field of Fat Studies builds on the reconceptualization and reclaiming of fat that has taken place in Fat Activism and the Fat Acceptance movement. We understand Fat Acceptance as a broad social justice movement which campaigns for the acceptance and appreciation of bodies of all sizes and shapes, and against the discrimination of fat people. In recent years, the Fat Acceptance movement has become increasingly active online. The use of the Internet is central in the increased visibility of Fat Activism. The online presence has improved connections between local activists, and has made local actions and individual projects accessible to broader audiences. One of the new modes of expression and political activism online that has been widely appropriated by Fat Acceptance is blogging. Kate Harding and Marianne Kirby, two prominent figures in the online community, estimate that the Fatosphere really took flight in the year 2007 (2009: 183). The term "Fatosphere," used for the online communities of fat activists and bloggers, is an ironic reference to the term "blogosphere" which is used for the blogging world in general. The fat bloggers form a *community* in the sense that they maintain close ties, engage with each other's posts and actively support each other.

While the Fatosphere (and online space in general) is a significant space for activism and community building, it is important to note that virtual reality online and digital technologies are closely related and shaped by the aforementioned mind/body split. Early cybernerds fostered a dream that virtual reality would be a space to escape and leave the "meat" behind, "download" the human mind directly into a computer (Moravec, 1988) and get rid of the body as an unnecessary burden. This positions cyberspace (or virtual reality—VR) as a distinct and ultimately different space, disconnected from the fleshy here-and-now altogether: the opposition of VR and "real life" (RL) becomes yet another dualism resonating with that of the mind/body split. Such an approach has been extensively criticized (*c.f.* Hayles 1999) as denying the unavoidable entanglement of matter and information, mind and body, form and content.

Leaving the body out of VR influenced the way in which the potentials of cyberspace were envisioned. The Internet has been (and to a large extent still is) seen as an alternative, anonymous space where one can create and live different identities, forge connections that defy physical boundaries and empower oneself through doing that (Hayles 1999). However, as early as 1995, Sherry Turkle aptly pointed out that even though users do have an option of creating alternative identities that do not correspond to their "real lives," they often choose not to (Turkle 1995). The body sneaks back into cyberspace through embodied differences and real-life structures of inequality that get transferred to virtual spaces. Thus the relationship between RL/VR is to be seen rather as a feedback loop: RL influences the kind of spaces and potential that are opened up by VR, and the latter in its turn affects how we live and experience "real life." They resonate, mix, yet do not quite overlap. So what happens to this being-in-the-world when bodies, and particularly fat bodies, go online to consume porn?

Fat Sex Online: Mediating the Flesh, "Meating" the Medium

Porn enters the discourses of VR as a sort of "clean sex" (Gillis 2004): it involves no exchange of bodily fluids with the performers on the screen—no need to touch or smell the other body—and social interactions are more easily controllable. And yet, pornography is all about the body. More than that: the body is its tool of address as well as its addressee. Pornography's aim is to make the body do and experience things. In that pornography aims at invoking physical reactions on the viewer's part, it falls into the category of "body genres": weepies (melodramas) and horror movies (Williams 1991).

Seen in this light, online pornography in itself is a counter-statement to the claim that the internet, and VR more generally, tend to disembody their users. Fat porn highlights corporeality even more by focusing on the excess of flesh. In a way we could say that online porn in general and fat porn in particular "meat" the Internet[2] and position the body and its carnality firmly at the core of mediated pleasure. Given the still prevailing mind/body dualism and implied hierarchy of thought and reason over flesh, excessive corporeality combined with network technology becomes an object of fascination in itself.

However, in the context of the Fat Acceptance movement, the question arises: what does fat porn do to and with "real" fat bodies and subjectivities and how much does it help or hinder the goals of Fat Acceptance? In our opinion, this question too often gets focused *only* on the issue of how much representations correspond to and influence reality. It seems to us that, at least in non-academic discourses, the assumption is often made that representations

2 We are borrowing this phrasing here from Maria Llopis' performance "Meat/ing the Internet," performed at Berlin Porn Film Festival in 2011. For more information see: http://www.mariallopis.com/en/portfolio/meating-in-the-internet/ (accessed June 12, 2013).

of fat bodies in porn have to "match" the lived reality of these bodies to be empowering, thus making representations a sort of "mirror images" of the lived fat experience. At the same time this assumption implies a particular model of "media effects": a model that, while claiming that images have effects on lived experiences, makes a clear distinction between the body (the effect) and the image (the cause) as defined, autonomous things and leaves out the importance of particular medium (Coleman 2012). This not only re-enforces dualistic models of thought, but also influences the kinds of strategies that can be employed in activist politics.

As an alternative to this kind of media effects model, Rebecca Coleman suggests that bodies and images are not separate but *become* through each other (2012). In her research of relations between bodies, images and experiences of teenage girls, she claims that: "[i]t is not, for example that images represent women—and should represent them better—but that, […] images make possible for women particular ways of seeing and knowing bodies. Bodies and images, then, are not separate but rather bodies are known, understood and experienced through images" (Coleman 2012: 19), and vice versa. In other words, what an image or representation can do to lived bodily experience depends as much on representation as it does on the body, and most of all it depends on the relations between them.

These relations, we argue, are those of dynamic and intensive experience of distance and closeness. These latter concepts are here to be understood as referring to the ability of the viewer to *relate* to what they see on screen, either by *recognizing* the representation as being in tune with their own experience, or by identifying with it without a shared experiential ground. This ability to relate is built on resonances between the image and the embodied viewer. However, "distant" images can be as affectively intense as "close" ones—they can shock, excite, disgust, and trigger a range of other emotional responses. As Susanna Paasonen explains, "[t]o resonate with one another, objects and people do not need to be similar, but they need to relate and connect to one another. Resonance encompasses the emotional and cognitive as well as the sensory and affective, and it points to the considerable effort involved in separating the two" (2011, p. 16). "Carnal resonance," according to Paasonen, involves "the viewers' ablity to recognize and somehow sense the intensities, rhythms and motions depicted in porn in their own bodies" (2014, p. 138). Thus there is a distinction to be made: while the distance and closeness describes the relation between the viewer and the image, "carnal resonance" is more of an affective quality of that relation. We argue further that carnal resonances are precisely what online porn attempts to create through visual means as well as discursive tropes, while the embodied viewers' experience of porn is more characterized by the notions of distance and closeness.

From Divas to Sluts: Tropes, Techniques and the Affective Grab of Online Fat Porn

One of the main questions that divided the feminist movement during the "sex wars" of the 80s was the question of what is the social impact of pornography and, related to the previous, what kind of purpose does it serve. The answer to this was closely related to the kinds of effects porn was thought to produce. The anti-porn feminists argued that pornography seduces by drawing on the existing material inequalities, such as those between the sexes, and thus reproduces the power dynamics that also result in material consequences, such as violence against women (Dworkin 1981). Anti-anti-pornography feminists responded to this line of argument by proposing that pornography is rather about fantasy and thus its effects cannot be as straight forward as anti-pornographers would suggest (Williams 1989). By now many more nuanced analyses of pornography's appeal have been developed. One of them is Paasonen's theory of the "grab." According to her, pornography attempts to *grab* the viewer through material-discursive means: porn appeals to the viewer's viscerality, to their bodly knowledge, but also discursive tropes and imagery related to them, notions of cultural value, taste and social hierarchies (Paasonen 2011, 256–8). In other words, porn tries to produce affective responses through visual and discursive techniques and it does that by foregrounding the excessiveness of the corporeal as well as power dynamics at play in society at large.

Consider, for instance, some of the titles from the Youporn.com BBW (Big Beautiful Women) category: "Huge Sexy BBW Gets Her Pussy Pounded," "Cock Hungry Huge Honey," "Thick Babe Fucked by Big Black Cock." Or some titles from RealBBWtube.com: "Fat Slut with Massive Tits Gets Licked," "Fat Slut Likes Skinny Cocks and Faces To Get Her Off," "Samantha 38G Dominates and Rides Amazon Skye Sinn," "Lovely Latina Jasmine Cox Fucks," "Watch Chubbie Boobies Bounce," "Ravishing Huge Tits," etc. These titles reflect social categories such as race ("latina," "big black cock") and gender ("slut"), and already connect them to the existing stereotypes related to these categories (racial stereotypes as in "*big* black cock," and gender stereotypes as in "*cock hungry* huge honey"). These titles are also constructed through excessive speech ("huge," "pounding," "massive"), and focus on carnality (specific body parts but also highlighting bodily actions or sensations such as hunger and fucking, for instance). Fat porn in particular further highlights the excess of the corporeal by focusing on the volume of flesh, often by foregrounding bodily differences ("fat slut" and "skinny cocks") as well as related power dynamics ("fat sluts" dominating or on the contrary—being "fucked" and overpowered).

The abundance of flesh is at the core of BBW porn imagery and discursive tropes used in it. Michael Goddard (2007) argues that it is precisely the volume of flesh that makes BBW porn performers into the figures of powerful women, privileged objects but also, and quite often, subjects of desire. If porn in general focusses on corporeality and portrays it in excess, in fat porn the excess of the corporeal is brought to the literal level in that it features bodies that would otherwise most likely be perceived as monstrous in more normative contexts. Both the discursive tropes that, according to Goddard, characterize fat porn—the fat woman as a Diva or Goddess, fat as the Dominatrix, the fat as the monstrous, the fat as craving for sex, the fat that has to be mastered and tamed[3]—as well as specific sexual practices, such as face sitting, the notorious practice of "pig hunting",[4] and feederism,[5]—reflect the attempt to grab the viewer's mind and body through playing with excess and power dynamics and their intertwinings. On the one hand, the fat body and its excessive corporeality in fat porn is meant to overwhelm, to overpower, and yet on the other hand the tropes of taming the unruly body, or of humiliation ("hunt down") are also quite prominent.

The excess is further increased through the very medium of the Internet and common architecture of "tube" websites.[6] The structure of tube websites meets the user with abundance of images, organized mostly in rows of frames, and tries to grab and hold their attention through both discursive (names of the videos, slogans and other textual material) as well as visual (flashing pop-ups and side-bar advertisements) means (Paasonen 2011). Thus we face a paradox, which is productive for online porn: on the one hand, online porn provides corporeality in excess, on the other hand it tries to manage that excess through categorization (into BBW porn, for instance).

The affective response that porn tries to produce by "grabbing" the viewer and the ability of the viewer to experience the images as distant or close, are not entirely unrelated. Certain forms of porn, and amateur porn in particular, are built on the assumption that seeing bodies and sex acts of "regular people" (as opposed to professional performers) creates an affective appeal that enables the viewer to relate to the image more easily. This not only has been shown in porn research that analyses amateur porn (for instance, van Doorn 2010) but manifests also in the way amateur porn is often proposed as connoting "realness" and somewhat

---

3 For more in-depth analysis of the roles, see, for instance, Goddard 2007 and Kipnis 1996.

4 "Pig hunting" or "hog hunting" refers to a practice usually exercised by a group of men who target fat women for sex, often as a joke. For more information see: http://en.wikipedia.org/wiki/Hogging_%28sexual_practice%29 (accessed June 12, 2013).

5 Feederism is a type of fetish practiced by people who derive sexual pleasure from (over)feeding. For more information see, for instance: http://bitchmagazine.org/article/feast-of-burden (accessed June 12, 2013).

6 We specifically refer here to the tube websites since they are the easiest way to gain access to various sorts of pornography for free, which makes them also the main contemporary gateway to pornographic imagery.

more "personal" approach. For example, user WetChubby on xHamster.com is ranked as a "porn lover," i.e. active porn consumer, and she also produced a video "Small masturbating video from me."[7] By tapping into the discourse of realness and handing over the production and performance to "laymen" with low skill and experience, amateur porn aims at bringing the virtual closer to the actual, "porn bodies" closer to "real bodies" and "real sex" (van Doorn 2010) thus suggesting that that which is "real" is somehow more affectively intense, more capable of creating resonances between the viewer and the image.

Online porn aims at "grabbing" the viewer through the use of both visual and discursive means. Furthermore, this "grab" is constructed by feeding from and back into different realms: mainstream porn culture, "realness" of amateurism, post/pseudo feminist discourse of empowered (and thus at the same time threatening) woman (Goddard 2007), the complex relation between reality and virtuality, production and consumption. The resulting tension thus creates multiple resonances that can produce effects of sexual gratification and disgust, feelings of empowerment and humiliation, the drive to put oneself "out there" through amateur porn or become a voyeur, etc. In other words, it is perhaps not so much about porn making bodies do things, but rather about dynamics of affective response and tapping into diverse contexts to invoke "carnal resonances" (Paasonen, 2011). These resonances encompass not only cultural production of fat porn and its different tropes, but also overspill into fat activism and lived fat subjectivities. In the next section, therefore, we will look at how the dynamics of distance/closeness and resonance operate in fat women's responses to fat porn.

Responses from the Fatosphere

In this section, we examine different points of view about fat porn that were sparked by the blogpost *Sex and the Fat Girl: The Joys of Fat Porn* which was posted on the Bitch website by guest-blogger Tasha Fierce on February 4, 2011. Bitch Media is the online presence of *Bitch Magazine*, a Portland-based feminist magazine founded in 1996 which presents itself as a "feminist response to pop culture" (http://bitchmagazine.org/history). With the series *Sex and the Fat Girl*, Tasha Fierce aimed to address topics related to fat acceptance and sexuality, such as attractiveness, insecurity, dating and (non)monogamy. In the first installment, Fierce explains the motivation for her series as follows: "I want to celebrate [fat sex], break down why there's such a barrier to discussing fat sex

7 Video available at http://xhamster.com/movies/1990632/small_masturbating_video_from_me.html and profile overview at http://xhamster.com/user/WetChubby (accessed June 12, 2013).

and critique the overarching societal values that seek to keep fat girls believing that they can't be sexual beings at the size they're at."[8] With this introduction, Fierce positions the series as a feminist and fat positive webspace, where norms around fat sex can be openly discussed.

We use the blogposts and the discussions that it opened up as a case study to illuminate different stances on fat porn that exist in an online feminist fat positive context. As such, the material of this specific case is not considered to be "representative" of a broader consensus within the online Fat Acceptance community. Indeed, there is no such consensus on the topic of fat porn; and there is no one viewpoint which could express all Fat Acceptance bloggers' take on fat and BBW pornography. Instead, we use the discussion to detect and analyze a variety of different responses and opinions that exist on the topic of fat porn within the online Fat Acceptance context.

As the title of the blogpost already indicates, the author Tasha Fierce is positive about fat porn, because she believes that it can "encourage people to see fat women as sexual beings" (Tasha Fierce). Speaking about her own experience, she writes that "I've found that watching porn with fat women in it to be a very good way to learn to appreciate and love your body, and to reinforce the idea that we are capable of enjoying sex as much as thin women" (Tasha Fierce). Her enthusiasm and positive feelings are shared by several commenters on the blogpost. For example, one commenter writes: "I love watching other big girls enjoy their bodies. It makes ME feel sexy. I feel like I am wanted" (Torria). Torria indicates that watching a fat body on the screen has the effect of making her own body feel attractive and desirable as well. Moreover, it is through seeing the performer enjoy her own body, that this feeling sexy and wanted comes about.

Fat porn is attractive to some commenters, because they feature "bodies like their own" and thus offer a point of recognition and relating. As one commenter expresses: "I automatically gravitate towards BBW porn because I like seeing bodies like my own. If I watch a thin girl in porn, I feel like I'm watching something I don't understand and I focus more on analyzing their bodies, which takes away from the point of porn for me" (artsykelly). Artsykelly here indicates that watching porn that features fat bodies makes it easier for her to relate to the images. Seeing a body like her own increases the familiarity; she feels closer to what she watches and is able to immerse herself in the experience. Conversely, watching videos featuring thin girls seems to have the opposite effect: a distance is created, and artsykelly finds herself analyzing the limbs and the bodies, losing the possibility to simply enjoy the scene. Watching fat porn *frees* her from the normative images of sex that are so far removed

8 See: http://bitchmagazine.org/post/sex-and-the-fat-girl-whats-it-all-about (accessed June 12, 2013).

from her lived corporeality. The images provided by fat porn are experienced by this commentator as being closer to her lived body and lived experience. Instead of having to imagine someone with a different type of body having sex, watching fat porn enables her to imagine her own body as a sexy and sexual body, and live that out. Of course, the question remains who the commenter Artsykelly relates to or identifies with in watching the porn video featuring fat bodies. Does she identify with the BBW performer, or does she identify with the desire *for* the BBW performer?

Other commenters do not feel empowered by watching fat porn, but rather associate it with feelings of insecurity and self-consciousness. Commenter Chris 77 writes: "I think fat porn would make me more self-conscious about my weight. Kind of a 'Oh, so that's what I look like … ' response. Currently the bedroom is one of the only places where I can strip off the stigma and judgments and just be the super sexy hotty my hubby treats me as" (Chris 77). Instead of feeling closeness, a distance is created precisely by seeing the images. "Knowing" what sex acts and positions look like from an outsider or third-person perspective creates a feeling of self-consciousness that hinders or even prevents altogether "being in the moment." Here, we can notice how the third-person perspective or *body image* affects the lived experience of sexuality, or *body schema.* It is interesting to note that the commenter indicates that this distancing seems to play a role both when watching pornography (the response "Oh, so that's what I look like"), *and* when having sex offline (taking the self-consciousness into the bedroom).

Other commenters voice a strong opposition to fat porn when they suggest that there is an explicit or implicit humiliating and degrading angle to pornography featuring fat bodies. An anonymous commenter writes: "I can see some feeling empowered by having a whole subsection of porn dedicated to their appearance, but it doubly hurts when another is visibly disgusted by it" (anonymous). The imagined response of other viewers is here postulated as being hurtful and wounding to fat people. This idea that anyone watching fat porn would be disgusted by it rather than turned on is graphically expressed by Goblyn: "I believe people view fat porn in the same matter that people view a train wreck—is it gross and [disturbing] but you cannot look away." Goblyn identifies herself as "a fat girl who loves porn," and does not indicate whether she herself shares the feelings that she so graphically describes. Her post seems to concern mainstream responses to fat porn, responses that nevertheless affect her as a fat girl living her sexuality. For these commenters, then, the imagined response of other viewers creates a distance to the image, which seems to be viewed as if through the eyes of another. Here, we again see a clear example of how the phenomenological distinction between *body image* and *body schema,* that was discussed above, collapses or disintegrates. The imagined response of others becomes central to one's own experience of the scene: the belief that others are disgusted by the image, profoundly colours and disturbs one's own appraisal of it.

In both these positive and negative evaluations of fat porn by the commenters on *Sex and the Fat Girl*, we can note that the respective empowerment or humiliation centers on a question of *identification* and *representation*: a supposed match between the fat body on the screen and the fat body watching the screen. Seeing a 'body like my own' is experienced by some as enjoyable and liberating, and by others as humiliating or degrading. While for some commenters, watching 'other big girls' enjoying themselves was empowering and enhanced their ability to see themselves as sexy and sexual subjects, for others this "likeness" was exactly disturbing, because it provoked thoughts of "Oh, so that's what I look like." It is clear that both the positive and the negative evaluations thus hinge on the same logics of 'mirroring' that we discussed earlier. The pornographic images serve as an image that either affirms or disrupts a certain self-perception.

Fat Porn as Stepping Stone or Roadblock on the Journey of Fat Acceptance

In many online and offline Fat Acceptance writings, Fat Acceptance is characterized as a "journey": a process which takes time and work. In *Lessons from the Fatosphere*, Kate Harding and Marianne Kirby write: "body acceptance does not come easily or all at once—it's a process. A long, slow process" (2007: 211). For many who embark on this journey it seems that *sexuality* is one of the 'hurdles' that must be faced and overcome. Dominant cultural ideas which equate fat with ugly and unattractive are pernicious and can be hard to shake off, even for someone who is active in Fat Acceptance and believes to have come to terms with their own fat body. This narrative which presents Fat Acceptance as an ongoing journey is very explicit in Tasha Fierce's blogpost on fat porn. Fierce speculates that an appreciation of fat porn could be seen as a *sign* of a more advanced and internalized fat acceptance: "Sometimes I wonder if the idea of fat/BBW porn is so disturbing to some because they're just not *there* yet. Maybe they're just not ready to accept fatness as sexy, maybe they're not far enough down that road—especially if they don't have a problem with porn with thinner people" (Tasha Fierce). Fierce here argues that a person who has 'truly' accepted her own fat would be able to appreciate fat porn, and that those who are disturbed by it have some way to go in their path toward a more complete self-acceptance and fat acceptance. A similar point is made by the commenter Susannah who writes:

> As a fatttie fat fat, and a sex-positive porn lover, I have to say that when I decided to come to terms with my body, I actively sought out BBW porn, erotica

> and art. Thousands of fatphobic comments required counteracting … I needed lots of fat adoration to beat back my ingrained self-hatred. I needed to see folks lick their lips in anticipation of jumping their jiggly partner, and hear the paeans to the loveliness of fat bodies before I could fully appreciate my own body. (Susannah)

Here, Susannah presents watching fat porn as a step in her own process of fat acceptance. We could even say that she presents it as a stepping stone: a way of furthering her own fat acceptance, bringing it to the next level. This is clear when she writes that *needed* to see these images, and *actively sought them out.* For her, they counteracted societal norms and discourses, and enabled her to fully appreciate her own body—in a way Susannah needed to tap into her own body image to accept the embodied reality of her body schema.

However, appreciation of fat porn does not necessarily need to be seen as a gage of internalized Fat Acceptance. Commenter Chris77 writes: "As a big girl with a great sex life who LOVES porn, this post struck a cord [sic]. I'll be buying porn today for V-day, and it will be decidedly skinny girl. Last night I sat up and wondered, 'Am I denying my own sexuality?' I don't think so." Here, Chris77 indicates that her interest in pornography featuring skinny girls should not be understood as a failure to accept her own fat. For her, the people in a porn video are not primarily bodies to identify or dis-identify with in regard to weight/size. Instead, she says "they are more of a personification of sexuality than actual people. Feeling any insecurity that I'm not as skinny as them is as ridiculous as my husband feeling insecure about not being as large as my vibrator" (Chris77). With these comments, Chris77 rejects the common narrative which sees fat porn as a necessary stepping stone for fat acceptance.

In the blogpost and the comments, participants also discussed whether there is necessarily an element of fetishization in fat porn or BBW porn. In her post, Fierce writes about different attitudes toward fat fetishism:

> I've heard fat girls say they think fat fetishism is creepy, that they feel objectified, that they feel the person with the fetish doesn't like them as a whole person … And that may all be true—except the creepy part, of course—but that doesn't mean that other fat girls don't enjoy engaging in fat fetishism and seek out people with said fetish, and it doesn't mean they are wrong for doing so. (Tasha Fierce)

Fierce argues that we should reserve judgment, and not condemn those who fetishize fat or those who enter into a relationship or sexual encounter with someone who fetishizes their fat. Erin Leigh responds by noting that she does take issue with some types of fat porn: "For me, what is important (in any porn, but especially with fat porn) is that there's a real sense of attraction and chemistry. Fetishization without respect is what feels creepy to me" (Erin Leigh).

An anonymous commenter who identifies as a Fat Admirer comments that finding fat beautiful and sexually arousing would not stop them from respecting and loving their fat partner (anonymous).

Other comments question the clear lines that Fierce seems to draw between a fetishistic and a non-fetishistic appreciation for fatness. An anonymous commenter writes "I have always loved [fat]/chubby girls for as long as I can remember. I don't consider it a fetish though. I also like redheads it isn't a fetish to be attracted to a body type or look. Is being attracted to white women a fetish or just what someone finds arousing?" (anonymous). Here, the line between "fetish" and simple "attraction" becomes blurred. Why is an interest in a fat sexual partner so often framed as a fetish instead of a preference? When is an interest in a particular body part/type rightly characterized as a "fetish," and what does that characterization do? Some commenters suggest that it is the intensity of the interest in fatness that could be seen as a decisive factor in distinguishing between fetishism and simple attraction. Other commenters argue that an interest in fat bodies is often associated with "fetish" because of the stigma which is still attached to the idea that "fat" can be sexy. Nikita writes: "Why are people who appreciate beautiful fat women's bodies considered 'weird' and 'objectifying'? I'm not some kind of weirdo!" (Nikita). Another anonymous commenter wrote: "I just wish we could get to the point where being sexually aroused by a fat person was no longer considered a fetish, but a preference" (anonymous).

In the discussion on fetishization, the underlying problem seems to be that a focus on specific body parts and bodily aspects is experienced as a lack of recognition of fat embodied subjectivity. Rather than being 'seen' as a living, breathing, thinking, feeling and desiring being, the fat person is reduced to *just* her flesh. Some commenters take issue with this compartmentalization and objectification of the body, through the focus on one particular aspect of the body, its fatness, because it may come at the expense of appreciating the full embodied subject. Other commenters consider this "objectification" a normal and regular part of sexual attraction, and argue that it is only because this particular type of sexualizing an aspect of embodied being is less common, that is perceived with suspicion.

Sex and the Fat Girl: The Joys and Sorrows of Fat Porn

The different responses to Tasha Fierce's blogpost *Sex and the Fat Girl: The Joys of Fat Porn*, showcase a variety of different opinions on fat pornography that were voiced in a fat positive feminist webspace. In our analysis, we have shown that some fat commenters have a very positive association with porn featuring fat bodies: they wrote about feeling empowered by seeing bodies like their own in a sexual context, and framed the viewing of fat pornography as a step in an ongoing process of increasing fat-/self-acceptance. Others expressed a more troubled relation to fat pornography; pointing attention to potential humiliating or degrading elements in the representations of fat women. The commenters wrote about how they individually as fat-bodied persons related to fat porn, and how it affected them physically and emotionally.

One difficulty with the discussion as a whole is that participants talked about "fat porn" without specifying what types of websites, genres or videos they had in mind. There was a tendency to discuss fat porn in a generic mode: as if it is "one thing." The diversity of different types of porn featuring fat bodies was not reflected in this discussion. When talking about fat porn as either degrading or empowering, different participants to the discussion could in fact have very different examples in mind.

One of the few distinctions that was made in the discussion, was a distinction between "queer porn" and "mainstream porn" featuring fat bodies. Commenter Jesse Dangerously and Erin Leigh reflected on the different representations of fat bodies in these types of fat porn. Erin Leigh believes that queer porn allows for more positive representations of fat bodies, and specifically mentions the website queerporn.tv as "a great example of how to feature chubby and fat bodies in a hot and empowering way" (Erin Leigh). While Jesse Dangerously agreed with this, she also argues that queer porn is not the *only* place where fat bodies should be visible and represented. According to her, "the queering of fat bodies and experience pretty much is what keeps them marginalized in the mainstream. Therefore, settling for body-inclusivity in queer contexts unfortunately challenges nothing about mainstreams perspectives on fat or other othered types of bodies" (Jesse Dangerously).

This discussion about the relative merits of queer fat porn vis-a-vis "mainstream" fat porn makes explicit a normative undercurrent that is typical for discussions around pornography and which seems to characterize this discussion as well. This normative undercurrent is an implicit or explicit desire by the participants in the discussion to characterize fat porn as something that is either good or bad; essentially empowering or degrading for fat women. Feeling themselves distanced by fat porn that does not resonate with their lived experiences of fat embodiment and fat sexuality, commenters distance themselves from these expressions.

This type of evaluation of the merits of pornography featuring fat bodies stays focused on the level of individual recognition and dis-recognition: the pornographic image as a mirror that either pleases or upsets. The central concern for many commenters seems to be whether the images in the scene properly match to their lived experiences of sexuality, their fat embodiment of sexual agency. If the images are found to be pleasing and empowering, this is because they are considered closer to reality, truthful to embodied fat sexualities that the commenter in question experiences. If the images are found to be disturbing, this is because they are seen to represent fat sexuality in a way that does not match the first-person experience of fat sexuality, disrupting the body schema through the body image that presses itself up and inhibits. In our view, this mode of evaluating the merits or problems of fat porn are legitimate. However, we consider the focus on "proper" and "truthful" representations to be somewhat limiting. While fat porn can and should certainly be judged on the level of representation, perhaps this is not the only level where we could evaluate it.

In our analysis, porn is not only about reality and a "match" with reality. As we have seen in the previous section, we see porn much more as a process of creating carnal resonances and the attempt to "grab" the viewer's attention and invoke bodily responses through excessive language, focus on carnality and exaggeration of power. Being supposedly "close to reality" is only one of the many means that pornography employs to achieve that. Seeing a "body like your own" can be empowering on an intellectual level but for many of the commenters we also saw that it was not the primary criterion for selecting porn.

Conclusion: Creating Resonances

In this chapter we showed that fat porn online is experienced by fat viewers through the dynamics of distance and closeness that are based on the resonances between lived body and the image. These resonances, however, are not only about the question of the ability of the viewer to relate to the pornographic image, or how well it corresponds to the way "real" fat women experience sexuality. They are also results of complex entanglements of discourses of porn culture, dis/embodiment in virtual reality, potentials of online spaces and web 2.0 culture, and experiences of (as well as discourses around) fat embodiment and empowerment. This renders online fat porn not so easily categorizable into "good porn" and "bad porn" (not least because it begs the question: bad/good for whom?) and invites us to think about fat porn and its use for fat activism without reducing complexities or trying to fix clear-cut standards.

One way to enact the political potential of fat porn can be through seeking representations that are more attuned to the experience of lived fat subjectivities. The responses on the *Sex and the Fat Girl* blogpost indicate that such "closeness" is currently not experienced by fat women and girls. Rather, some feel a distance because of degrading and humiliating elements. Amateur trends in porn can be a means and a space for alternative productions, opening up the possibility to create porn that is close to lived experiences of sexuality.

However, one has to be wary of the pitfalls that the labels "reality" and "amateurism" can create, namely the fixing of what counts as a "real" experience of sexuality and a "true" representation of it. We would like to suggest that there are also other promising directions: instead—or perhaps rather "next to"—looking at how much representations and realities match, fat porn can be a realm for experimentation with one's sexuality. As fat porn performer April Flores puts it:

> I feel very lucky that I have had the chance to explore and expand my own sexuality through my work in pornography. I have lived out my own fantasies … I've been able to experience many scenarios … These opportunities have led me from identifying as a straight woman to understanding that my sexuality is fluid and not dictated by the gender of my partner. (Flores 2013: 281)

Without ascribing normative value to queer sexualities, we see the potential in exploring pornography as a space to perform and experiment. If pornography is more about resonances than straight-up representation-reality match, then the political potential lies in looking for creative languages for sexual expression that acknowledge the variety and complexity of lived experiences and the multiple ways that they are shaped. Thus finally, to relate back to Coleman's idea that bodies and images become through each other, we would like to encourage people to ask not only whether pornography featuring fat bodies should properly and truthfully *represent* the lived experience of fat subjects, but also whether the affective resonances that these images invoke enable fat women to live their sexualities in a more fulfilling and empowering way.

References

Bordo, S. 2003. *Unbearable Weight.* 2nd edition. Berkeley: University of California Press. (Original work first published 1993).

Coleman, R. 2012. *The Becoming of Bodies: Girls, Images, Experience.* Manchester: Manchester University Press.

van Doorn, N. A. J. M. 2010. *Digital Spaces, Material Traces: Investigating the Performance of Gender, Sexuality, and Embodiment on Internet Platforms that feature User-Generated Content.* Amsterdam: UvA Universiteit van Amsterdam.

Dworkin, A. 1981. *Pornography. Men Possessing Women.* London: The Women's Press Ltd.

Fierce, T. 2011. Sex and the Fat Girl: The Joys of Fat Porn, in *Bitch Magazine.* [Online]. Available: http://bitchmagazine.org/post/sex-and-the-fat-girl-fat-porn [June 12, 2013].

Flores, A. 2013. Being Fatty D: Size, Beauty, and Embodiment in the Adult Industry, in *The Feminist Porn Book: The Politics of Producing Pleasure*, edited by

Tristan Taormino, Celine Parreñas Shimizu, Constance Penley and Mireille Miller-Young. New York: The Feminist Press: 279–83.

Gillis, S. 2004. Cybersex, in *More Dirty Looks. Gender, Pornography and Power*, edited by Pamela Church Gibson. London: BFI Publishing: 92–101.

Goddard, M. 2007. BBW: Techno-archaism, Excessive Corporeality and Network Sexuality, in *C'Lick Me. A Netporn Studies Reader*, edited by Katrien Jacobs, Marije Janssen and Matteo Pasquinelli. Amsterdam: Institute of Network Cultures: 187–96.

Hayles, N. K. 1999. *How We Became Posthuman: Virtual Bodies in Cybernetics, Literature and Informatics*. Chicago, London: University of Chicago Press.

Hemmings, C. 2005. *Invoking Affect: Cultural Theory and the Ontological Turn, Cultural studies*, 19(5): 548–67.

Kipnis, L. 1996. *Bound and Gagged: Pornography and the Politics of Fantasy in America*. New York: Duke University Press.

LeBesco, K. 2004. *Revolting Bodies? The Struggle to Redefine Fat Identity*. Amherst, MA: University of Massachusetts Press.

Levin Russo, J. 2007. 'The Real Thing': Refraiming Queer Pornography for Virtual Spaces, in *C'Lick Me. A Netporn Studies Reader*, edited by Katrien Jacobs, Marije Janssen and Matteo Pasquinelli. Amsterdam: Institute of Network Cultures: 239–52.

Merleau-Ponty, M. 2002. *A Phenomenology of Perception*. (Smith, C., Trans.). New York: Routledge Classics (original work first published 1945).

Moravec, H. 1988. *Mind Children: The Future of Robot and Human Intelligence*. Cambridge, MA; London: Harvard University Press.

Mowlabocus, S. 2007. Gay Men and the Pornification of Everyday Life, in *Pornification: Sex and Sexuality in Media Culture*, edited by Susana Paasonen, Karina Nikunen and Laura Saarenmaa. Oxford, New York: Berg: 61–72.

Murray, S. 2008a. Normative Imperatives vs. Pathological Bodies, *Australian Feminist Studies*, 23(56): 213–24.

Murray, S. 2008b. *The "Fat" Female Body*. New York: Palgrave Macmillan.

O'Toole, L. 1998. *Pornocopia. Porn, Sex, Technology and Desire*. London: Serpent's Tail.

Paasonen, S. 2011. *Carnal Resonance: Affect and Online Pornography*. Cambridge, MA: MIT Press.

Paasonen, S. 2014. Between Meaning and Mattering: On Affect and Porn Studies, *Porn Studies*, 1(1–2): 136–142.

Smith, C. and Atwood, F. 2013. Emotional Truths and Thrilling Slide Shows: The Resurgence of Antiporn Feminism, in *The Feminist Porn Book: The Politics of Producing Pleasure*, edited by Tristan Taormino, Celine Parreñas Shimizu, Constance Penley and Mireille Miller-Young. New York: The Feminist Press: 41–57.

Tischner, I. *Fat Lives: A Feminist Psychological Exploration*. Sussex: Routledge.

Turkle, S. 1995. *Life On Screen: Identity in the Age of the Internet.* New York: Simon & Schuster.

Welton, D. 1998. *Body and Flesh: A Philosophical Reader.* Malden: Blackwell.

Williams, L. 1989. *Hard Core: Power, Pleasure and the "Frenzy of the Visible."* Berkeley: University of California Press.

Williams, L. 1991. Film Bodies: Gender, Genre, and Excess, *Film Quarterly*, 44 (4): 2–13.

Young, I. 2005. *On Female Body Experience: 'Throwing Like a Girl' and Other Essays.* Oxford: Oxford UP.

Creative Interlude

Chapter 10
Dumpling

Alison Winch

She presses her belly against the hob
and drops balls of broken dough,
strung out and held in nets. The water is furious.
She watches so they don't turn sad,
so they swell to rhizomes,
and then she lets them sit, tied up and resting.

Upstairs, she searches for a silky
thing of bone
to make a waist; she hooks and knots,
she holds her breath, lifts her ribs,
creates a shape, and pulls –
the figure stays: *bait.*

She stands to eat the dumplings
steamed to diamonds. Her silhouette shifts and digs.

Culturally (In)visible Bodies

Chapter 11
Amy Lowell's Appetites: Food, Consumption and Homoerotic Desire in Amy Lowell's Poetry

Sarah Parker

Introduction

Few early twentieth-century writers have suffered such a dramatic fall from favour as Amy Lowell. Between 1912 and 1927, Lowell published 11 volumes of poetry (including three posthumous collections edited by her life-long companion Ada Dwyer Russell), edited three volumes of Imagist verse (*Some Imagist Poets*, 1915–1917) and played a central role in promoting and defending the 'New Poetry' in America. By 1922, she was 'regarded as a "national institution" whose slow and laboured approach to a speaker's lectern was the signal for the audience to rise' (Ruilhley, 1975, p. 141). She also used her wealth and influence, as a member of the famous Boston Lowell family, to financially support and encourage other significant modernist poets, including H. D., Richard Aldington, and D. H. Lawrence. At the time of her death, Amy Lowell was one of the most prolific and successful poets of her time; a revered American 'woman of letters' who graced the cover of *Time* Magazine in March 1925, just months before her death. She had recently completed yet another daunting project; a two-volume biography of John Keats. A transatlantic lecture tour was planned – a trip that Lowell, sadly, never took, due to her death from a sudden stroke at the age of 51.

But despite her many achievements, a year later, the project of deriding and eventually forgetting Amy Lowell, was already underway. In 1926, Clement Wood published *Amy Lowell*, a barely veiled attack on the poet, which criticised her work as corrupted by her perverse desires (he complained that her love lyrics: 'do not word a common cry of many hearts') and willed her to disappear from cultural memory: 'We have much that, for Miss Lowell's sake, must be forgotten, and will be' (p. 173, p. 96). He also notes that '[h]er bodily frame was excessively stout and ungainly' (p. 31) and perpetuates the rumour that her alleged self-disgust led her to demand that 'every large mirror … be swathed in black' (p. 33). This book was just the beginning of a series of so-called critical studies that denigrated Amy Lowell's considerable achievements, using her wealth, sexuality and body as weapons against her. Such biased portrayals culminate in Hugh Kenner's *The Pound Era* (1973), which dubs Lowell 'the hippopoetess' (a term coined by Lowell's enemy, the poet Witter Bynner) and describes her 'crossing like a big blue wave' to greedily 'appropriate' the Imagist movement 'since she had not been properly accepted' (p. 292).

Nonetheless, Lowell refused to disappear altogether from literary history. One fact about her remained, to be consistently repeated: the fact that Amy Lowell was fat. This fact might appear irrelevant in comparison to Lowell's innovative poetic output and vigorous support of modernist movements. But though her size has frequently been used to condemn and undermine her, it has also enabled Lowell to survive as a persistent presence in accounts of literary modernism. She lives on in bitchy biographical anecdotes: the fat woman as butt of the joke. Adrienne Munich and Melissa Bradshaw, editors of the essay collection *Amy Lowell: American Modern*, concede that: 'It is her corpulence … (not her considerable literary contributions) that have kept Amy Lowell in literary memory' (2004, p. xxiii). Lowell's size, as far as her survival in literary history is concerned, has therefore proved to be both her blessing and her curse.

For this reason, Lowell provides an interesting and provocative focus for fat studies. Her life narrative and subsequent critical denigration (in terms that condemn both her fat body and queer sexuality) combines the concerns of both fat studies, literary studies, gender and queer studies. The project of reclaiming Lowell as a fat woman recalls Elena Levy-Navarro's work on the seventeenth-century poet and playwright Ben Jonson. Levy-Navarro argues that observing historical figures such as Jonson, who reconceptualises his weight in terms of his integrity and worth as a friend, can offer us 'a model of how a fat history can use the past to speak to the predicament of the present … The past helps us reinterpret our fat in ways that are transformative' (p. 21).[1] As with the reclamation of queer histories, Levy-Navarro claims that 'we should come to see how [historical] figures who are defiantly fat speak directly to the present in ways that can sustain us' (p. 20).

Amy Lowell certainly qualifies as such a figure. Lowell flaunted her fat body at a moment when the very associations of fatness were shifting from positive to negative: from a sign of prosperity to a marker of greed, laziness, and even criminality. As Laura Fraser notes, whilst earlier in the nineteenth century 'a man with a thick gold watch swaying from a big, round paunch was the very

1 For example, Jonson, who was attacked in his own day for being fat, humanises 'weight' as a positive quality, writing: 'First weigh a friend, then touch, and try him too' (qtd. In Levy-Navarro, 2009, p. 21).

picture of American propriety and vigor ... Between the 1880s and 1920s, that pleasant image of fat thoroughly changed in the United States' (2009, p. 11). By the end of the nineteenth century, the European fashion for slenderness had taken hold. The shift from agricultural to industrial economies meant that even the poorest people were less likely to go hungry – being fat was therefore 'no longer was a sign of prestige' (Fraser, 2009, p. 12). Simultaneously, as women's roles shifted away from the home and into the public sphere, the fashion for thinness intensified; by the 1920s, the stream-lined, boyish figure of the flapper had become associated with forward-thinking modernity, in contrast to the now passé and regressive figure of the fat woman.

Into the midst of this hostile environment marched Amy Lowell, whose body and behaviour visibly defied the expectations placed on American women during both the late-nineteenth and twentieth centuries. Lowell provoked scandal by smoking cigars in public; she lived extravagantly and unapologetically, co-habiting with a beloved female companion, and she did all this in a body which was defiantly fat. Moreover, through her live poetry readings, Lowell implicitly insisted that a connection be drawn between her body and her words, as the site and expression of pleasure. For example, the poem 'Bath' (from her poem-cycle 'Spring Day', 1915) revels in the sensual enjoyments of the body in the bathtub: 'I lie back and laugh, and let the green-white water, the sun-flawed beryl water, flow over me' (*Men, Women and Ghosts*, 1955, p. 145).[2] The connection was too much for some to handle: Lowell's live reading this poem at the annual meeting of the Poetry Society of America in 1915 led to outrage: 'because of her very bulk the effect of it was almost as shocking as if she had actually appeared in her bathtub in public' (Gould, 1975, p. 174). Some accounts even claim that audience members angrily charged the podium after Lowell's performance.

Both Lowell's body and her poetry defied the strict dictates of avant-garde modernism, which favoured a hard, concrete, pared-down aesthetic. Lowell was attacked by Ezra Pound for usurping the Imagist movement; he then dismissed the movement as 'Amygisme', condemning the 'mushy technique' and 'floppiness' of Lowell's poetry (qtd. in Bradshaw, 2004, p. 172). These terms suggest the fluidity and softness of the fat female body, which Pound also reviled, attacking Lowell both through public insults and in letters to his friends and associates. Pound's criticisms of Lowell's work recall what Leslie Heywood has defined as the 'anorexic aesthetic' of modernism:'[i]n both the high modernist artist and the anorexic there is a rejection and a will to eliminate the feminine ... to shape the "base material" into a "higher", masculine form' (Heywood, 1996, p. 61). Therefore, the modernist emphasis on 'hardness, paring down, and reducing the poetic body can be read as a corollary for the ...

2 *Men, Women and Ghosts* (1916) will be hereafter referenced as *MWG*.

reduction or elimination of the female body' (Heywood, 1996, p. 101). With her fat body and her prolific poetic output, Lowell threatened to overwhelm the boundaries of Pound's neatly chiselled Imagism.

The reputation of Lowell's work and the pejorative connotations attached to the fat body are therefore intrinsically linked, affecting Lowell's reputation during her lifetime and her posthumous reception later in the twentieth century. However, given that Lowell's poetry has received limited critical attention in comparison with her peers (such as H.D.), we might argue that analysing Lowell's corporeality is a distraction, preventing us from paying much-needed attention to her work. However, there is much to be gained from interrogating how Lowell chose to display, construct, conceal, or perform her own embodiment as a fat woman. In her extensive scholarship on Amy Lowell's body, Melissa Bradshaw argues that Lowell often used her bulk to her advantage, to announce her presence and to help her to promote her work. Surveying a range of biographies which cast Lowell as a tragic victim of a 'glandular disorder', Bradshaw concludes: 'Missing from the ubiquitous descriptions of Lowell's body is any sense of joy it may have given her, any sense that she believed in its integrity, in the rightness of her embodiment' (2011, p. 44). Such joy can, for instance, be detected in Lowell's poem 'Bath'. In contrast to portraits of Lowell as the victim of an obesity that robbed her of any pleasure in her fleshliness, in this poem Bradshaw argues: 'the body that soaks leisurely in the bathtub … avow[s] the materiality of [Lowell's] experience and the erotic pleasures associated with that' (2004, p. 182).

My chapter aims to re-read Lowell's *poetry* in light of Bradshaw's suggestive comments, exploring 'the pleasure [Lowell] takes in physicality' (Bradshaw, 2011, p. 45). I want to examine closely the connections between food, appetite and eroticism in Lowell's poetic work – looking at how Lowell frequently uses food imagery as a metaphor for sexual pleasure, and appetite as a metaphor for desire. We can see this especially in Lowell's most famous volume *Pictures of the Floating World* (1919), which contains love lyrics inspired by her relationship with her lifelong companion Ada Russell. This volume features numerous examples of cooking and eating; from the 'baked white cakes' of 'Interlude' to the honey, wine and baked bread of which symbolises 'A Decade' with her partner. It is worth noting here that my attempt to identify and reclaim the sensual pleasures of eating in Lowell's poetic work in a sense works against the aims of fat studies scholarship, which often seeks to move away from notions of blame and culpability and associations of the fat body with excessive eating and 'the individual's lack of control' (LeBesco, 2004, p. 30). However, in the spirit of Levy-Navarro's call for an imaginative reclamation of past 'figures who are defiantly fat' (2009, p. 20), I want to present Lowell as a fat woman who revelled in her appetites, as a queer icon who was multiply transgressive, who defied attempts to apologise for or rehabilitate her stubborn body, and who insisted on the fat body as both the site and product of sensual pleasure. Ultimately, I argue that Lowell's celebration of the sensual enjoyments of cooking and eating reaffirms both the pleasure she took in her embodiment as a fat woman, and the *jouissance* of same-sex eroticism that she experienced in her relationship with Russell.

Dining with Amy Lowell

Amy Lowell's voracious appetite and love of food is evident from her letters and biographical studies. One particular anecdote from her childhood crops up repeatedly in biographies, as the apparent 'root' of Lowell's 'obesity'.[3] This story is originally recounted in S. Forster Damon's comprehensive *Amy Lowell: A Chronicle* (1935):

> It was when she was eight years old ... that she went to a party, where a large plate of rice was set before her. Her brother dared her to eat a second plate – she did – but when they prepared to go home, her coat would not button across her stomach. 'And it never buttoned again', Miss Lowell said, describing the episode. It was the first manifestation of her physical maladjustment. (p. 51)

Despite this episode attesting to Lowell's considerable appetite, and her determination not be outdone by her brother, the final sentence also demonstrates how Lowell biographies often attempt to blame Amy Lowell's 'obesity' on a glandular problem or 'chemical imbalance', in order to absolve her of any charges of 'greediness' or responsibility for her condition. These insistent medical interpretations projected onto Lowell's body by her biographers reflect the twentieth-century tendency to pathologise fat as a disease, to portray the fat individual as a pitiable victim, and to seek to 'cure' the fat body – a tendency today manifested in the search for the 'fat gene', which, as Kathleen LeBesco observes, worryingly echoes the late-nineteenth and early twentieth-century eugenicist theories surrounding homosexuality (LeBesco, 2009).

Another Lowell biographer Jean Gould, builds a contradictory picture of a rapacious Lowell and the indulgent upper-class society in which she moved,

3 I use the problematic term 'obesity' (see Wann, 2009, pp. xi-xii) consciously here, to indicate the way in which Lowell's biographers repeatedly interpret her fat body in pathologising, medicalised terms – for example, as the result of a chemical imbalance, a glandular 'problem' or as a manifestation of psychological trauma. Melissa Bradshaw provides a comprehensive survey of these anti-fat biographical attitudes in 'Remembering Amy Lowell: Embodiment, Obesity, and the Construction of a Persona' (2004).

but again concludes that glandular problems were to blame for Lowell's weight: 'Amy Lowell had always had a large appetite and loved to eat; one look at the menu of a typical dinner party of the day makes one wonder why the entire upper-class population did not suffer from obesity as Amy did ... It was obvious that her trouble was glandular, but most doctors believed the cure lay in diet alone' (1975, p. 67). Recounting the brief (and disastrous) episode in which Lowell, in her early twenties, tried a drastic 'reducing' diet pioneered by Dr William Banting (which involved travelling down the Nile, while surviving on a diet of asparagus and tomatoes), Gould however admits that: 'Amy Lowell was never one to do anything by halves. She was a person of extremes, and now ... she gave way indulgently to all the foods she loved' (1975, p. 72). Try as they might to ignore or downplay it, Lowell's biographers keep encountering the fact that Lowell clearly enjoyed eating and – with the exception of the Egyptian trip – never tried to reduce her food intake during her adult life, despite being fully aware that she was fat.[4]

Unsurprisingly, food and dining played a central role at Lowell's home of Sevenels. Lowell's dinner parties, hosted with the intention of bringing together the diverse writers, artists, composers and actresses that she particularly admired, are legendary. Lowell shared her life at Sevenels with Ada Dwyer Russell, a former character actress, who became Lowell's lifelong partner (and sometime amanuensis) from 1914 onwards. Together, the two women worked out a daily routine that suited their preferred lifestyles and fostered Lowell's creative work. Lowell preferred to write throughout the night and sleep through the day, so Russell ran the household during the daytime, trying to preserve as much quiet as possible. In the evening, guests would be received by Russell, and Lowell would join the dinner party half-way through the meal, having just risen from her bed. Damon describes a typical Sevenels dinner party in detail:

> The dinner was an old-fashioned one, with oysters, soup, fish, meat, salad, dessert, and fruit, accompanied (until Prohibition) with the appropriate wines ... then the meal continued, while the vanished courses reappeared, miraculously

4 Lowell's awareness of her weight, and her carefree enjoyment of eating are both revealed in a letter to her friend Eleanor Robson Belmont, thanking her for her gift of Sherry's chocolates: 'Your bounty is beyond words, and the worst of it is that I have, with the most meagre assistance, eaten it all up. I have been afraid to weigh myself since the deed was – Ah, but I do like Sherry's chocolates! ... The joy is only so much enhanced because it partakes of the nature of forbidden fruit. With every delectable drop, I feel a pound going on, and only when I recollect how short is life, how fleeting, do I reflect that it makes very little different whether a skeleton was once fat or thin. This consoles me greatly, and I eat on, unmoved and unmoving' (qtd. in Gould, 1975, p. 330).

> fresh, for Miss Lowell's consumption. Although she usually had two plates of soup and was always the center of the conversation, the dessert was served almost simultaneously. Then, after peppermints and ginger were passed, the party proceeded into the geniality of the library. (1935, p. 265)[5]

Following the meal, Lowell would lead the conversation whilst puffing away on one of her famous cigars. Damon writes that 'The flavour of those conversations can never be communicated … She could talk brilliantly on any subject' (1935, p. 265). At 11 o'clock, Ada Russell would ensure that a cold supper tray was set out, ready for Lowell's consumption during the night as she wrote. Guests would depart just after midnight, ready to catch the last car to Boston at 12.15.

From this brief description, we can observe the ways in which Lowell and Russell's relationship dynamic resembled that of a conventional husband and wife. Russell ran the household, whilst Lowell was engaged in the 'business' of poetry. Though Russell did not actually undertake the cooking and cleaning herself, she did manage Lowell's considerable staff, including cooks, servants and typists. Lowell's vast wealth (inherited through the Lowell family's cotton mill businesses) meant that food at Sevenels functioned as a sign of social power and conspicuous consumption, with Russell performing a role akin to 'lady of the manor' or society hostess. Occupying a position akin to the 'lord of the manor', Lowell clearly dominated the social gatherings at Sevenels, engaging in fierce discussions with (usually male) writers and artists, often her rivals. In this sense, the division of labour within Lowell and Russell's relationship can be compared to that of the modernist writer Gertrude Stein and her partner Alice B. Toklas. Together for 39 years, Stein and Toklas considered themselves 'married' and used the epithets 'husband' and 'wife'. But as Catherine R. Stimpson notes: 'the marriage was Victorian. The bluffer, bigger, more athletic Stein could do more, think more, say more … The tinier, more ladylike Toklas was more restrained … As Gertrude talked with the men … Alice talked to the wives' (1984, p. 130). This dynamic reflects Lillian Faderman's observation that professional women of the early twentieth century 'had no need for a husband but plenty of need for a wife' (1981, p. 213) – frequently, a close female companion fulfilled this role. Sandra Gilbert and Susan Gubar also note that modernist women writer's creative enterprises were often joint achievements, with one partner gaining most recognition for what was, essentially, collaborative work. It is interesting to note that such unequal relationships are represented via differences in body size; Stimpson describes a 'bigger' Stein and a 'tinier' Toklas, associating the

5 We can find evidence of Lowell's frequent social gatherings in 'The Dinner Party' (*MWG*, 1955, p. 146), a sequence of short poems in which a hostile social discussion takes place across six different courses, 'Fish', 'Game', 'Drawing-Room', 'Coffee', 'Talk' and 'Eleven O'Clock'.

fat female body with certain masculine freedoms (to 'do more, think more, say more') in contrast to the comparative feminine 'restraint' of the thin body.

Despite their same-sex relationship, Stein and Toklas's domestic and professional life was therefore still divided along gendered lines, with one partner adopting the 'masculine' role of artist/genius, the other the 'feminine' role of caregiver and homemaker. One of the most obvious ways in which this dynamic played out was in terms of cooking and eating: 'Stein ate, and Toklas cooked and served. Such acts, which Toklas taught herself to do magnificently, were literally and symbolically nourishing' (Stimpson, 1984, pp. 129–130). Stein clearly valued Toklas's ability to conjure up delicious meals, whilst Toklas found that her culinary abilities gave her a degree of power and influence in the household of this 'genius'. Though Stein employed professional cooks (demonstrating the ways in which socioeconomic power shaped this same-sex relationship), Toklas's gastronomic contributions demonstrated her support and devotion to her partner in the early days of their relationship, and ensured that she became indispensable. Later in life, in *The Alice B. Toklas Cookbook* (1954), Toklas reflected on her early forays in the kitchen, which – tellingly – coincided with the beginnings of her relationship with Stein:

> Before coming to Paris I was interested in food but not in doing any cooking. When in 1908 I went to live with Gertrude Stein on the rue de Fleurus she said we would have American food for Sunday-evening supper … the servant would be out and I should have the kitchen to myself. So I commenced to cook the simple dishes I had eaten in the homes of the San Joaquin Valley in California – fricasseed chicken, corn bread, apple and lemon pie. Then when the pie-crust received Gertrude Stein's critical approval I made mince-meat and at Thanksgiving we had a turkey. (2004, p. 29)[6]

Food also took on a symbolic role in the Stein-Toklas union. In Stein's writings, food and eating are used to represent desire. For example, in 'Lifting Belly', Stein puns flirtatiously: 'Here is a bun for my bunny. / Every little bun is of honey. / On the little bun is my oney. / My little bun is so funny' (qtd. in Gilbert and Gubar, 1989, p. 243).[7] Stein's speakers often adopt the roles of 'husband' or 'baby' – both of whom need to be fed by a doting mother/ wife; a role fulfilled by Toklas. Stein's voracious 'baby', as Sandra Gilbert and Susan Gubar note 'frequently asks to eat or be eaten, to please or be pleased'

---

6 Stein also recounts Toklas's discovery of cooking in *The Autobiography of Alice B. Toklas* (1933), in this case adopting Alice's voice: 'I like cooking, I am an extremely good five minute cook, and beside, Gertrude Stein liked from time to time to have me make American dishes' (Stein, 2001, p. 124).

7 Stein's *Tender Buttons* (1914) also contains an entire section entitled 'Food'.

(1989, p. 243). Thus, erotic and gastronomic appetites are conflated in Stein's work, and the lines between self and other become increasingly blurred. In a psychoanalytical sense, Stein might be said to have received a kind of pre-Oedipal gratification from indulging in repetitious, rhythmical language and by consuming the mother's body – her work dramatises a kind of Semiotic banquet. In Lowell's poetry too, we find that the pleasures derived from food and sex are collapsed together, reflecting Lowell's enjoyment of her fat body, in defiance of the intensifying cultural dictates that insisted both fat bodies and homoerotic desires should be yoked with guilt, denial and self-hatred.

Wine, Berries and Almonds: Consumption and Desire in Lowell's *Sword Blades and Poppy Seed*

As with Stein, we can find ample evidence of Lowell's enjoyment of food and eating in her poems. For example, the 'Bath' poem from Lowell's 'Spring Day' sequence is followed by a poem which celebrates the sensory joy of the 'Breakfast Table': 'the rolls of bread spread themselves in the sun to bask. A stack of butter-pats, pyramidal, shout orange through the white ... Coffee steam rises ... The day is new and fair with good smells in the air' ('Breakfast Table', *MWG*, 1955, p. 146).[8] Lowell repeatedly uses food imagery in her poems, from the sensuous, overripe fruits of 'Market Day' (*A Dome of Many-Coloured Glass*, 1912) to the Impressionistic 'Thomson's Lunch Room – Grand Central Station: Study in Whites':

> Jagged green-white bowls of pressed glass
> Rearing snow-peaks of chipped sugar
> Above the lighthouse-shaped castors
> Of grey pepper and grey-white salt.
> Grey-white placards: "Oyster Stew, Cornbeef Hash, Frankfurters" ...
> Two rice puddings and a salmon salad
> Are pushed over the counter. (from 'Towns in Colour', *MWG*, 1955, pp. 149–150)

As we can see here, food represented an ideal opportunity for an Imagist poet such as Lowell. Food items provided the Imagist poet with strong, definite images that can be presented in themselves, yet described in such a way that

8 Lowell's breakfast, would, of course, have been enjoyed in the afternoon rather than the morning, due to her unconventional timetable (thank you to Helen Hester for pointing this out to me). This poem may therefore be an exercise of imagination, as with the poem 'Interlude' (analysed later in this chapter) when Lowell describes baking cakes.

they resonate with deeper significance. Lowell's presentation of this lunchroom table, with this sugar bowls and salt castors, can be likened to the still life of Post-Impressionist painting (e.g. a Cézanne or Van Gogh) in which motionless objects take on the character of emotional states.

In Lowell's early work, food and drink often symbolise both erotic pleasure and the torment of unsatisfied desire. Several of the love lyrics published in Lowell's second volume *Sword Blades and Poppy Seed* (1914) associate desire with sensations of hunger and satiety. These poems were written when Lowell was trying to convince Russell to live with her. The two women met briefly in 1909, and again in 1912, but Russell continued to tour with her acting troupe, only staying with Lowell during the summer months. Lowell repeatedly asked her to come and live at Sevenels as her permanent companion (in June 1914, Russell finally relented). Lillian Faderman suggests that 'it is possible to conjecture Lowell's emotional state during these years from the apparently autobiographical poems' of *Sword Blades*, which present the speaker as 'imploring, apologetic, and entirely at the mercy of the beloved who … is depicted as goddess, mother, healer, and holder of the sole and elemental power to rescue the speaker from alienation and pain' (2004, p. 59, p. 60).

A number of short lyrics in *Sword Blades* employ the motif of the overflowing wine-cup to represent the speaker's thirst for the beloved, and the intoxicating effects of quenched desire.[9] In a longer narrative poem entitled 'The Shadow' (SB, 1955, pp. 66–71), Lowell also connects the consumption of food and drink to physical tangibility and the possibility of fulfilled desire. 'The Shadow' is a fable that draws on elements of the Pygmalion myth: a poor watchmaker, Paul Jannes, toils to complete a watch for a wealthy customer. Working through the night, Paul becomes infatuated with what appears to be the shadow of a woman cast upon the wall: 'No woman was in that room! … / What made / That beautiful, dreadful thing, that shade / Of something so lovely' (1955, p. 67). After offering the shadow an array of jewels and other gifts, Paul comes to believe that *feeding* the shadow will bring her into tangible existence: 'Man grows by eating, if you eat / You will be filled with our life, sweet / Will be our planet in your mouth. / If not, I must parch in death's wide drouth' (1955, p. 70). The items Paul buys for this banquet – bread and wine – have Eucharistic significance. He watches over the baking bread: 'As rapt-souled monks watch over the baking/ Of the sacred wafer' (p. 70). But this holy communion is really an anticipation of erotic communion, as Paul hopes that eating will substantiate the shadow with a physical body:

9 See for example the following poems in *Sword Blades and Poppy Seed* (1914): 'Absence' (p. 41), 'A Gift' (p. 41), 'Anticipation' (p. 42) and 'Vintage' (p. 42).

... Red as blood
Was the wine which should bring the lustihood
Of human life to his lady's veins ...
He put meat on her plate and filled her glass,
And waited what should come to pass. (1955, p. 70)

The shadow, alas, remains a shadow, and Paul commits suicide from grief and disappointment. This poem, however, is significant for the connection it draws between nourishment and sexual fulfilment: here, Lowell places the body and its tangibility at the centre of her poem, explicitly connecting the act of eating with the act of making love. Lowell later returned to Eucharistic imagery in her poem 'In Excelsis' (1927); a poem that connects consumption with lesbian erotic communion.

In addition to the brimming wine-cup and Eucharistic imagery, another key image of consumption in *Sword Blades and Poppy Seed* is that of ripe fruit, particularly berries. Lowell had already described delicious fruits in an earlier poem, 'Market Day' in which 'bartering booths spread out their tempting shows / Of globed and golden fruit, the morning air / Smells sweet with ripeness ... / A wicker basket gapes and overflows / Spilling out cool, blue plums' (*A Dome of Many-Coloured Glass* [1912], 1955, p. 20). Lowell's language here recalls Christina Rossetti's *Goblin Market* (1862), in which fiendish goblins offer two innocent sisters an array of tempting fruits: 'Apples and quinces, / Lemons and oranges, / Plump unpeck'd cherries, / Melons and raspberries, / Bloom-down-cheek'd peaches' (2008, p. 67). *Goblin Market* has frequently been read as a metaphorical fable about female sexuality, the 'forbidden fruit' recalling Eve's eating of the apple in the Garden of Eden.[10] Ripe fruit also represents the fecundity of the fertile female body. Isobel Armstrong describes *Goblin Market* as a 'deeply, insatiably oral poem' (1993, p. 348), both in terms of its subject-matter and its repetitive metre/rhyme scheme. The same could be said of Lowell's poem 'The Fruit Shop' (from 'Bronze Tablets'), in which a pushy fruitseller rhythmically promotes his succulent wares:

And those grapes! They melt in the mouth like wine,
Just a click of the tongue, and they burst to honey.
They're only this morning off the vine ...
Those oranges – Gold! They're almost red.

10 See, for example, influential readings by Margaret Homans, '"Syllables of Velvet": Dickinson, Rossetti, and the Rhetorics of Sexuality (*Feminist Studies* 11, 1985, pp. 569–593) and Cora Kaplan, 'The Indefinite Disclosed: Christina Rossetti and Emily Dickinson' in *Women Writing and Writing about Women*, ed. Mary Jacobus (New York: Barnes & Noble, 1979), pp. 61–79.

They seem like little chips just broken away from the sun itself. Or perhaps instead
You'd like a pomegranate, they're rarely gay,
When you split them the seeds are like crimson spray. (*MWG*, 1955, p. 111)

The pomegranate image appears again in Lowell's poem 'Miscast II'. The speaker, bursting with unfulfilled desire, declares:

My heart is like a cleft pomegranate
Bleeding crimson seeds
And dripping them on the ground.
My heart gapes because it is ripe and over-full,
And its seeds are bursting from it. (*SB*, 1955, p. 42)

The image of the 'cleft pomegranate' is strikingly erotic, suggesting a wet, glistening opening, and the ripeness of the fruitful womb. We find a similar image in a fin-de-siècle poem by Michael Field entitled 'Unbosoming' (1893):

The love that breeds
In my heart for thee!
As the iris is full, brimful of seeds,
And all that it flowered for among the reeds
Is packed in a thousand vermilion-beads
That push, and riot, and squeeze, and clip,
Till they burst the sides of the silver scrip (1893, p. 84)[11]

Though one poem concerns a pomegranate and the other an iris, both poems utilise the image of seeds bursting out of a heart overflowing with passion. Noting that references to small, round objects such as seeds, nuts and buds recur in nineteenth-century women's poetry, Paula Bennett has suggested that such imagery can be read as clitoral symbolism: 'identifying their "little hard nut[s]" – or their little flowers – with "something precious", women are expressing … their conscious or unconscious awareness of the organic foundation of their (oxymoronic) sexual power'– oxymoronic in the sense that the clitoris is 'little' yet 'tremendous force [is] nevertheless contained within it' (1990, p. 172, p. 173).[12] Examples of clitoral imagery listed by Bennett include 'peas, pebbles,

11 'Michael Field' is the collaborative pseudonym of Katharine Bradley and Edith Cooper, an aunt and niece who considered themselves 'closer married' than the Brownings.

12 Bennett notices such clitoral imagery is particularly prevalent in Emily Dickinson's work. It is worth noting that Emily Dickinson is mentioned in Lowell's most famous poem 'The Sisters' (1925) as a key female precursor.

beads, berries, nuts, buds, crumbs, pearls, pellets, dews, gems, jewels, drops, and … bees' (1993, p. 236).

Small, round objects such as seeds, berries and nuts feature heavily in Lowell's love lyrics, evoking not only Lowell's own female embodiment, but also her homoerotic desires. It is significant that these objects are all *edible*, suggesting an oral eroticism at play in these poems. This eroticism that comes most clearly to the fore in Lowell's poem 'Aubade':

> As I would free the white almond from the green husk
> So would I strip your trappings off,
> Beloved,
> And fingering the smooth and polished kernel
> I should see that in my hands glittered a gem beyond counting. (*SB*, 1955, p. 73)

Here, Lowell uses the simile of unshelling an almond to describe undressing the beloved.[13] The poem printed before 'Aubade', entitled 'White and Green' also addresses the naked beloved as an almond: 'You are an almond flower unsheathed / Leaping and flickering between the budded branches' (p. 73). In 'Aubade', love-making is implied through the reference to tenderly 'fingering' the 'smooth and polished kernel'. The comparison of this small, smooth almond to a 'gem' only underscores the clitoral symbolism in this poem. A later poem, 'The Weather-Cock Points South' (*Pictures of the Floating World*, 1919), employs similar symbolism, though this time Lowell describes a flower-bud:

> I put your leaves aside,
> One by one:
> The smooth, broad outer leaves;
> The smaller ones,
> Pleasant to touch, veined with purple;
> The glazed inner leaves.
> One by one
> I parted you from your leaves,
> Until you stood up like a white flower
> Swaying slightly in the evening wind. (1955, p. 211)

Faderman identifies the flower image here as a 'descriptive symbol for female genitalia' and the act described as cunnilingus – suggested by the 'breath' of the wind on the flower (2004, p. 73). Such imagery, crucially, enabled Lowell to write about lesbian love-making without attracting censorship – something

13 Gould recounts how Lowell once 'told a shy young poet that unwrapping her little Manila [cigar] was like undressing a lady' (1975, p. 119).

she experienced indirectly through her friend D. H. Lawrence, whose novel *The Rainbow* was banned in 1915, in part due to a lesbian love scene.

As with her notorious public reading of 'Bath', Lowell subtly draws attention in her poetry to her corporeality as a fat woman and her homoerotic appetites. One of ways she achieves this is by associating homoerotic desire with a *flavour*: an appetite for almonds in Lowell's work ultimately comes to stand in for homoerotic desire and lesbian identity. For example, in a later poem entitled 'To Two Unknown Ladies' (published posthumously in *Ballads for Sale*, 1927), Lowell considers her response to Somerville and Ross (Edith Somerville and Violet Florence Martin) – nineteenth-century women writers whose close relationship and collaboration paralleled that of 'Michael Field' (see footnote 11). Reading their work, Lowell is unaccountably 'haunted' by these two dead spinsters: 'I go back to you again, / Evening and evening, in a kind of thirst, / Surprising my tongue upon an almond taste' (1955, p. 563). The significance of the almond flavour is never explained within the poem, though it is reaffirmed later on: 'Almonds, I said, / Smooth, white, and bitter, wonderfully almonds' (p. 564). If we read this poem in light of Lowell's oeuvre then this 'moment of recognition' becomes clear (Donaldson, 2004, p. 38). Through their veil of their writings, Lowell spies the story of Somerville and Ross's intimate relationship; a close companionship that parallels her and Russell's: 'Two lives which stare and twinkle on the page / So that I blind in looking' (p. 565). Lowell provocatively figures this recognition of lesbian sexuality through taste – the flavour of almonds upon the tongue. Rather than being ashamed of her embodiment *or* her sexuality, Lowell's poetry covertly celebrates and affirms such transgressive appetites.

The Domestic Goddess: Ada Russell in *Pictures of the Floating World*

In 1914, Ada Russell finally agreed to become Lowell's permanent companion. Her presence in Lowell's household can be detected throughout the series of love lyrics that Lowell published in *Pictures of the Floating World* (1919), particularly the section entitled 'Two Speak Together'. *Pictures* has repeatedly been cited as Lowell's most successful collection of love poems: Paul Lauter dubs it 'the most fully articulated sequence of lesbian poetry between Sappho and the 1960s' (2004, p. 5).[14] The volume is consistently associated with Russell as Lowell's lesbian muse, a biographical reading supported by the fact that Lowell wanted to dedicate the volume to her partner (Russell refused to grant permission for such a public acknowledgement). The poem also features specific details

14 For more on Lowell's love poems in *Pictures*, see Faderman (1981, 2004) and Gilbert and Gubar (1989).

of domestic life at Sevenels, including the presence of Lowell's dogs and the extensive garden which forms the setting for many of the poems.

Though Russell, unlike Alice B. Toklas, did not actually cook for her partner, she does repeatedly appear in the guise of a kind of 'domestic goddess' in *Pictures*, undertaking household tasks such as baking, gardening and sewing. For example, in 'Madonna of the Evening Flowers', the absent beloved is represented by: 'your books, / … your scissors and thimble just put down' (1955, p. 210). She eventually appears in the garden: 'Standing under a spire of pale blue larkspur, / With a basket of roses on your arm' (p. 210). She gives the speaker a series of gardening instructions: 'You tell me that the peonies need spraying, / That the columbines have overrun all bounds, / That the pyrus japonica should be cut back and rounded' (p. 210). In 'A Sprig of Rosemary', Lowell depicts the beloved's hands, engaged in domestic tasks:

> I cannot see your face.
> When I think of you,
> It is your hands which I see.
> Your hands,
> Sewing,
> Holding a book,
> Resting for a moment on the sill of a window. (*Pictures*, 1955, p. 216)[15]

In another poem entitled 'Interlude', Lowell's speaker describes the baking and decorating of cakes:

> When I have baked white cakes
> And grated green almonds to spread on them;
> When I have picked the green crowns from the strawberries
> And piled them, cone-pointed, in a blue and yellow platter;
> When I have smoothed the seam of the linen I have been working;
> What then?
> To-morrow it will be the same:
> Cakes and strawberries,
> And needles in and out of cloth. (*P*, 1955, p. 212)

I suggest that in this particular poem, Lowell actually adopts Russell's voice, in a comparable way to Gertrude Stein's ventriloquism of Alice B. Toklas. The daily domestic tasks described in the first half of the poem are more reflective of Russell's household role than Lowell's. As we know, Lowell kept to a strict

15 Lowell's focus on the beloved's hands recalls the important role of hands and fingers in lesbian eroticism (see Blain, 1999, p. 137).

routine of sleeping all day, and writing all night, so the day-time setting of the first half of the poem is more suited to Russell's timetable than Lowell's. Add to this the fact that Lowell was useless at household tasks and 'abhorred' needlework and the activities described at the beginning of 'Interlude' become less applicable to the poet herself and more an imaginary account of her partner's day.

Margaret Homans is the only critic to note that the speaker of 'Interlude': 'might be Ada addressing Amy (since the actual Amy probably never prepared food or sewed a seam), or the poem might represent a dialogue' (2001, p. 336). As I have argued elsewhere, Lowell's ventriloquism of Russell has a number of problematic implications – this seizure of another's voice can be read as an act of appropriation, silencing her female partner in order to foster her own creative expression. Gilbert and Gubar, for example, read Gertrude Stein's *The Autobiography of Alice B. Toklas* (1933) in this way: 'Usurping Alice's persona, appropriating Alice's voice, Stein … turns collaboration into collusion … the result is a kind of cannibalism, as Stein makes Alice into a character of her own devising' (1989, p. 251). It is interesting that these critics use the metaphor of consumption to signify such an appropriation of voice and identity – pejoratively linking this appropriation to the aggressive hunger of the fat lesbian body. But despite her apparent 'cannibalism' of Russell in 'Interlude', elsewhere Lowell demonstrates an anxious awareness of the ethical issues implicated in speaking for, or as, another woman – for example, in the two-part poem 'Anecdote' (*Ballads for Sale*, 1927) she voices both the male poet and the female muse, who stands, naked and objectified: 'Why do you strip me before all these people / … are you so cynical that you expose me for a whim?' (Lowell, 1955, p. 577). 'Anecdote' reveals Lowell's anxious awareness that the masculine position of suppliant she occupied in many of her poems was predicated on a power-imbalance that sapped agency from the female muse whilst ostensibly exulting her and occasionally appropriating her voice.[16]

Whichever way we interpret it, what is perhaps most striking about Lowell's poem 'Interlude' is the careful sensuality with which the speaker describes her actions – spreading, arranging, smoothing and moving her needle in and out of cloth. The (previously discussed) almond image and 'cone-pointed strawberries' add to the subtle eroticism of this poem, meaning it functions doubly; as a delicate description of home-making and a covert celebration of love-making. In her later poems, Lowell increasingly appeals to religious imagery, particularly the Eucharist, to celebrate her physically and spiritually nourishing relationship with Russell. The transformation of bread and wine into Christ's body and blood for Lowell comes to represent the transformative

16 For an expansion of this argument, see Sarah Parker, *The Lesbian Muse and Poetic Identity, 1889–1930* (2013), 'Amy Lowell' chapter.

effects of her relationship. This is clearly seen in 'A Decade', a poem which marks ten years after meeting Russell:

> When you came, you were like red wine and honey,
> the taste of you burnt my mouth with its sweetness.
> Now you are like morning bread,
> Smooth and pleasant.
> I hardly taste you at all for I know your savour,
> But I am completely nourished. (*P*, 1955, p. 217)

Returning here to the wine symbolism of *Sword Blades*, Lowell describes the change in her relationship. Russell has become the wholesome daily bread, rather than burning wine of passion. Desire – and the pain of absence – has now been replaced by contentment and commitment. Lowell affirms that though long-term companionship may lack a strong flavour, it nonetheless nourishes 'completely'.

These religious metaphors assert themselves most strongly in a triad of poems in the posthumously published *What's O'Clock* (1927). These poems inspired by the structures of Roman Catholic liturgical worship are entitled 'Prime' (morning prayer), 'Vespers' (evening prayer) and 'In Excelsis'. The latter poem – its title deriving from the Latin hymn 'Gloria in Excelsis Deo' ('Glory to God in the highest') – depicts the beloved as a fertility goddess who brings abundance with her every step:

> You – you –
> Your shadow is sunlight on a plate of silver;
> Your footsteps, the seeding-place of lilies;
> Your hands moving, a chime of bells across a windless air.
> The movement of your hands is the long, golden running of light from a rising sun;
> It is the hopping of birds upon a garden-path. (*WOC*, 1955, p. 444)

Once again, floral imagery is abundant here: the beloved's fertility-giving powers are emphasised by the 'seeding-place' of lilies; she is later compared to 'the perfume of jonquils' (p. 444), a member of the Narcissus family and 'the flower symbolic of falling in love with likeness' due to their growing by water (Vanita, 1996, p. 51). Lowell uses metaphors of pollination to describe the beloved's inspirational powers: 'Your words are bees about a pear-tree, / Your fancies are the gold-and-black striped wasps buzzing among red apples' (p. 444). In 'The Poem', the speaker is completely reliant on the beloved to plant and water her 'green bud' (*P*, 1955, p. 227). This image recalls an earlier poem in *Pictures*, 'Flame Apples' which is an extended metaphor for the creation of poetry:

Little hot apples of fire,
Burst out of the flaming stem
Of my heart,
I do not understand how you quickened and grew.
And you amaze me
While I gather you. (1955, p. 226)

Images of fruit and bees thus provide a metaphor that combines the quickening of creativity with sexual fulfilment. In 'April', this culminates in a kind of birth:

I will lie under the beech-trees …
In a blueness of little squills and crocuses.
I will lie among the little squills
And be delivered of this overcharge of beauty,
And that which is born shall be a joy to you
Who love me. (*P*, 1955, p. 213)

In 'In Excelsis', Lowell again utilises Eucharistic images, as the beloved is consumed by the speaker, filling her as water fills an empty vessel:

I drink your lips,
I eat the whiteness of your hands and feet.
My mouth is open,
As a new jar I am empty and open.
Like white water are you who fill the cup of my mouth (*WO*, 1955, p. 444)

The speaker represents herself as 'jar' and 'cup', recalling wine-cup of *Sword Blades*. But in earlier poems such as 'Absence' and 'A Gift', Lowell's speaker figures herself as a vessel that fills for the beloved: masochistically giving her blood and her words 'for your drinking' until she risks running dry (1955, p. 41). In 'In Excelsis', the roles are reversed: the speaker is nourished by the 'white water' pouring from the beloved's lips like milk from a mother's breast. This lesbian union is figured as a restorative feeding, revealing the intimate connection that Lowell draws between food and eroticism; pleasures experienced through her fat body. The empty fervour of wine is replaced by wholesome, life-giving milk. The nourishment pouring from the beloved's lips in 'In Excelsis', like her 'ripening' words, strengthens the speaker so that she can sing an ecstatic song of praise: 'I say 'Glory! Glory' and bow before you / As to a shrine/ … I take you, / I live' (p. 445). The poem itself – and, as Lowell later stated, *all* her poems – was the result of Russell's nurturing presence.[17] The final lines confirm this: 'those things I say in consequence / Are rubies mortised in a gate of stone' (p. 445). The ruby, set in stone, can be read as an image of the permanence of poetry: the speaker and the beloved will perish, but the beloved's beauty will be immortalised ('mortised') in the form of the poem. The 'gate of stone' also hints at the immanence of death – lending an extra poignancy to the fact Lowell's poem was published posthumously in a volume edited by Russell.

Conclusion

This chapter has shown that food played a number of important roles in Lowell's work. In Lowell's early love poems, particularly *Sword Blades and Poppy Seed*, hunger and thirst represent unsatiated desire. The over-flowing wine cup is used to signify the excesses of longing, which leads to desperation and a loss of self-control. Food items such as berries, almonds and seeds here (and elsewhere) function as clitoral symbols, enabling Lowell to allude to lesbian love-making without risking censorship. In the later love poems of *What's O'Clock*, the domestic goddess, sewing in the garden or baking, represents Russell, Lowell's beloved companion, and the life they shared together at Sevenels. The religious imagery of the Eucharist represents the sustenance Lowell received in this long-term relationship, culminating in the ecstatic praise-poem 'In Excelsis'.

Though a necessity at Lowell's time of writing, metaphorical descriptions of love-making and the female body later became an established convention of lesbian love poetry. For example, in *Twenty-One Love Poems* (1977), Adrienne Rich describes: 'your lovemaking, like the half-curled frond / of the fiddlehead fern in forests / just washed by sun' and 'your strong tongue and fingers / reaching where I have been waiting years for you / in my rose-wet cave' (1993, p. 83). Indeed, such imagery became so established that it took on the status of cliché. A 1981 drawing by cartoonist Jo Nesbit depicts a female folk singer announcing: 'I will now sing a short song comparing my lover's clitoris to a pearl, and her labia to a persimmon fruit and her vagina to a vanilla pod because quite frankly that's the only way I can cope with it all' (reprinted in Hennegan, 2000, p. 330). As Antje Lindenmeyer writes: 'The connection between food and sex can be a cliché … the suggestive shapes and textures of fruit lend themselves very easily to this' (2006, p. 471). But, as Lindenmeyer also shows, for contemporary lesbian writers such as Jeanette Winterson, Dorothy Allison, Audre Lorde and Anna Livia, food continues to carry a symbolic weight. In novels such as Winterson's *Oranges Are Not The Only Fruit* (1985) and Lorde's

17 Lowell was finally able to dedicate one book to Russell. The dedication to the *John Keats* (1925) biography reads: 'To A. D. R. / This and all my books / A. L'.

Zami (1982): 'Food is seen as integral to lesbian existence, intimately connected to and involved in the shaping of sexual identities, personal histories and lesbian communities' (Lindenmeyer, 2006, p. 482). Lowell's work is in many ways provides the foundation for this. Flying in the face of the biographies that cast her as a tragic victim of a 'glandular imbalance', Lowell's poetry expresses her radical, unashamed enjoyment of food, and affirms the delicious eroticism and sustaining fulfilment she experienced in her lifelong relationship with Russell.

References

Armstrong, I., 1993. *Victorian Poetry: Poetry, Poetics and Politics*. London: Routledge.

Bennett, P., 1990. *Emily Dickinson: Woman Poet.* Hertfordshire: Harvester Wheatsheaf.

——, 1993. 'Critical Clitoridectomy: Female Sexual Imagery and Feminist Psychoanalytic Theory', *Signs: Journal of Women in Culture and Society*, 18.2, pp. 235–259.

Blain, V., 1999. 'Sexual Politics of the (Victorian) Closet; *or*, No Sex Please – We're Poets'. In: I. Armstrong and V. Blain (eds), *Women's Poetry, Late Romantic to Late Victorian, Gender and Genre, 1830–1900.* London: Macmillan.

Bradshaw, M., 2004. 'Remembering Amy Lowell: Embodiment, Obesity, and the Construction of a Persona'. In: A. Munich and M. Bradshaw (eds), *Amy Lowell, American Modern.* New Brunswick, New Jersey and London: Rutgers University Press, pp. 167–185.

——, 2011. *Amy Lowell: Diva Poet.* Farnham: Ashgate.

Damon, S. Foster., 1935. *Amy Lowell: A Chronicle, with Extracts from her Correspondence.* Boston: Houghton Mifflin.

Donaldson, E. J., 2004. 'Amy Lowell and the Unknown Ladies: The Caryatides Talk Back'. In: A. Munich and M. Bradshaw (eds), *Amy Lowell, American Modern.* New Brunswick, New Jersey and London: Rutgers University Press, pp. 27–42.

Faderman, L., 1981. *Surpassing the Love of Men: Romantic Friendship and Love between Women from the Renaissance to the Present.* London: The Women's Press.

——, 2004. '"Which, Being Interpreted, Is as May Be, or Otherwise": Ada Dwyer Russell in Amy Lowell's Life and Work'. In: A. Munich and M. Bradshaw (eds), *Amy Lowell, American Modern.* New Brunswick, New Jersey and London: Rutgers University Press, pp. 59–76.

Field, M. 1893. *Underneath the Bough.* London: George Bell and Sons.

Fraser, L., 'The Inner Corset: A Brief History of Fat in the United States'. In: E. Rothblum and S. Solovay (eds), *The Fat Studies Reader.* New York and London: New York University Press, pp. 11–14.

Gilbert, S. M., and S. Gubar, 1989. *No Man's Land: The Place of the Woman Writer in the Twentieth Century. Volume Two: Sex Changes*. New Haven: Yale University Press.

Gould, J., 1975. *Amy: The World of Amy Lowell and the Imagist Movement.* New York: Dodd, Mead & Company.

Heywood, L., 1996. *Dedication to Hunger: The Anorexic Aesthetic in Modern Culture.* California: University of California Press.

Homans, M., 2001. 'Amy Lowell's Keats: Reading Straight, Writing Lesbian', *The Yale Journal of Criticism*, 14.2, pp. 319–351.

Kenner, H., 1973. *The Pound Era.* California: University of California Press.

Lauter, P., 2004. 'Amy Lowell and Cultural Borders'. In: A. Munich and M. Bradshaw (eds), *Amy Lowell, American Modern.* New Brunswick, New Jersey and London: Rutgers University Press, pp. 1–8.

LeBesco, K., 2004. *Revolting Bodies? The Struggle to Redefine Fat Identity.* Amherst and Boston: University of Massachusetts Press.

——, 2009. 'Quest for a Cause: The Fat Gene, the Gay Gene, and the New Eugenics'. In: E. Rothblum and S. Solovay (eds), *The Fat Studies Reader.* New York and London: New York University Press, pp. 65–74.

Levy-Navarro, E., 'Fattening Queer History: Where Does Fat History Go from Here?' In: E. Rothblum and S. Solovay (eds), *The Fat Studies Reader.* New York and London: New York University Press, pp. 15–22.

Lindenmeyer, A., 2006. '"Lesbian Appetites": Food, Sexuality and Community in Feminist Autobiography', *Sexualities*, 9. 4, pp. 469–485.

Lowell, A., 1955. *The Complete Poetical Works of Amy Lowell.* Boston: Houghton Mifflin.

Munich A., and M. Bradshaw, 2004. 'Introduction'. In: A. Munich and M. Bradshaw (eds), *Amy Lowell, American Modern.* New Brunswick, New Jersey and London: Rutgers University Press, pp. xi–xxvi.

Parker, S., 2013. *The Lesbian Muse and Poetic Identity, 1889–1930.* London: Pickering & Chatto.

Rich, A., 1993. '(The Floating Poem, Unnumbered)'. In: B. Charlesworth Gelpi and A. Gelpi (eds), *Adrienne Rich's Poetry and Prose.* New York: Norton, p. 83.

Rossetti, C., 2008. *Selected Poems.* London: Penguin.

Ruilhley, G. R., 1975. *The Thorn of a Rose: Amy Lowell Reconsidered.* Connecticut: Archon Books.

Sappho, 1994. *Greek Lyric I: Sappho & Alcaeus* (Loeb Classical Library), Trans. D.A. Campbell. Cambridge, Massachusetts and London: Harvard University Press.

Stein, G., 2001. *The Autobiography of Alice B. Toklas* (1933). London: Penguin.

Stimpson, C. R., 1984. 'Gertrice/Altrude: The Paradox of the Happy Marriage'. In R. Perry and M. Watson Brownley (eds), *Mothering the Mind: Twelve Studies of Writers and Their Silent Partners.* New York: Holmes and Meier, pp. 122–139.

Toklas, A. B., 2004. *The Alice B. Toklas Cook Book* (1954). London: Serif.
Vanita, R., 1996. *Sappho and the Virgin Mary: Same-Sex Love and the English Literary Imagination*. New York: Columbia University Press.
Wann, M., 2009. 'Foreward: Fat Studies: An Invitation to Revolution'. In: E. Rothblum and S. Solovay (eds), *The Fat Studies Reader*. New York and London: New York University Press, pp. ix–xxv.
Wood, C., 1926. *Amy Lowell*. New York: Harold Vinal.

Chapter 12
Coming of Age through Weight Loss: The Fat Woman as Sexually Amature in Margaret Atwood's *Lady Oracle*

Michelle Green

The fat woman in Western fiction, culture and scholarship is half myth and half human. At her most potent and powerful, the fat woman is a goddess—Venus herself—with abundant, giving flesh that inspires readers, writers and scholars alike. At her lowest, she is not quite there at all—a sad, invisible figure laden with a body that leaves her alienated from the social world. These extremes of character are the recognizable "types" of the fat subject, a figure relegated to the fringe of "normal." However, the fat woman is both and always hypersexed and asexual. The othering of fat sexuality is not a binary but a continuum that is shifting, fluid and interdependent.

It is the commonalities within the representation of fat women's sexuality that inspires my contribution to this discussion. Through Margaret Atwood's third published novel *Lady Oracle* (1976) this chapter will examine the complex interchange between abjection, de-sexualization and the subjectivity of the fat woman as she ages from child to adult. Set in post Second World War Toronto, Ontario, *Lady Oracle* offers one of the first interrogative critiques of this dissonant position by following the life of Joan Foster, the 240 pound protagonist. A coming of age story, it explores Joan's experience as a chubby child, to a fat adolescent, and finally to a slim, nomadic traveller as she accumulates several secret lives that become harder to maintain. As the novel progresses it tracks the unconventional methods Joan uses to establish her own selfhood against her mother, society, and the lovers she takes. Joan's body remains central to the novel as a site of expression, destruction and self-creation originating in Joan's tense childhood relationship with her mother and culminating in her final act of defiance as she fakes her own death. An accidental poet and a writer of gothic costume romances, Joan's fractured sense of self leaves her spiralling into a self-destructive path in which fiction and reality collapse.

Atwood's *Lady Oracle* pre-dates other novels that use weight loss to signify psychological change, such as Carol Dawson's southern family saga *Body of Knowledge* (1993), Jennifer Weiner's chick lit *Good in Bed* (2001) and Frances Kuffel's weight loss memoir *Passing for Thin* (2004), and critiques the illusionary ideal behind weight loss rhetoric that is predicated on "new body, new life." While Atwood positions weight loss as formative in Joan's coming of age story she also provides an oblique criticism of weight loss as positively transformative through Joan's psychological collapse and struggle for subjectivity.

Through *Lady Oracle* this chapter will examine the fat heroine's othering and its relationship with "sexual amaturity," a term I use to refer to the negation of a character's social and sexual maturity. Through Joan Foster, I argue sexual amaturity is the state of being "out of sync" with reproductive and social time that renders the heroine afflicted by an oscillating childlikeness and pre-mature spinsterhood in society. From this, I establish weight loss as a formative experience similar to a re-birth or "coming of age" and argue *Lady Oracle* is the first in a series of weight loss coming of age novels. In this trend weight loss positions the fat woman "in sync" with her age and socially visible as a sexual being. As a form of social, sexual and even political awakening, the bodily transformation of the fat heroine functions as a socially formative experience similar to marriage in traditional female *bildungromans* (a subgenre of the masculinist coming of age novel that tracks the maturation of a single protagonist). I argue the weight loss coming of age novel should be read as a subset of this subgenre. Finally, in establishing the significance of weight in experiences of gender, sexuality and adolescence I conclude with an examination of how the weight loss novel renegotiates feminist concepts of girlhood and biological conceptions of adolescence.

By positioning weight loss as formative, if not transformative, *Lady Oracle* adapts key tropes of the *bildungsroman*. The *bildungsroman*, otherwise identified as the novel of development and the coming of age story, came to prominence in the English language through writers such as Charles Dickens although it has since undergone many transformations. It typically depicts the education of the hero, an often naïve subject, as his passionately held ideals are gradually worn away through encounters into society which necessitates a more or less resigned acceptance of the social order. The weight loss coming of age novel is one such transformation of this genre with the protagonist's key transition appearing in the shift from fat to thin. In transitioning between embodied states, weight loss affirms the protagonist's acceptance of the social order through their new normativity, and signifies a "coming of age" and "new birth" through personal and social transformation. However, while taking key formulaic elements from the *bildungsroman*, I use the term coming of age because it opens up more room for interpretation. The *bildungsroman* will always denote a historically-located, euro-centric genre that is perhaps unhelpful when discussing texts that are now nationally, culturally and historically alienated from this geopolitical moment.

However, the weight loss novel also challenges traditional definitions of "coming of age" and the expected gratification of this social and biological process, which, as Kenneth Millard has argued, is to reach "full legal adult status" regarding cultural markers like "alcohol, sexual consent, driving license, marriage" (2007, pp. 4–5). In the weight loss novel this definition is shown to be hollow through the fat character's ability to move through cultural spaces through "passing" as older than their years, and therefore transgress legal barriers normally applicable for adolescents. Instead, the transformation of the fat character is entangled with perceptions of sexual maturity and their emergence as a cited/sighted sexual and gendered subject in society. Much like the female *bildungsroman*, which as Rita Felski argues necessitates a burgeoning political awareness, this awakening ushers in the character's consciousness of sex difference. In re-entering the social world after a significant weight loss the newly-thin character conforms with society's standards, finding themselves accepted, but simultaneously develops a heightened sense of identity disjuncture that makes the change ambiguous and often unrewarding.

There are three significant implications of reading weight loss as a coming of age experience. The first is, if weight loss is read as a process of maturation and sexual maturation then it also poses a radical challenge to linearity as it offers multiple experiences of maturation, as well as multiple projections of self. Atwood explores in *Lady Oracle* that a subject may be socially unrecognized as of a sexually mature age despite biological sexual development. It may be possible for a character to experience more than one coming-of-age life narrative within the same novel. *Lady Oracle*'s protagonist Joan Foster is an example of how experiences of maturation on an individual, social and gendered agent can *run parallel* and *conflict*, *suppress*, and *contradict* each other.

The second implication is the breadth of texts that can be included and interrogated in this framework drastically expands. One such inclusion would be narratives of aging in which the aged body is perceived to digress into childlikeness or immaturity, as mentioned previously. I read both adolescence and aging as complex categories that denote both a biological and post-pubescent position and a socially constructed position that responds to sociological and psychological *ideas* of maturity. Viewing maturity as unfixed and unstable allows for a rich interrogation of its meaning and a re-examination of the coming of age genre, which provides room for aging narratives that turn on a similar "awakening."

Finally, this reading suggests a new comparative discourse for scholarship on adolescence and Atwood studies. While scholarship has already moved away from the biological in concepts of adolescence, favouring its psychological and sociological significance, there is more room for a comparative discourse with post-menopausal temporality. To open up Rachael McLennan's definition of adolescence, amaturity is also "experiential" as an "indeterminate and ambiguous period of existence negotiated by young people" and old persons, who may or may not identify with these categories, and "theoretical, a category variously informed by and resisting various disciplines such as psychology and sociology" (2013, p. 109). Adopting a more inclusive lens that looks at ages outside of reproduction complements scholarship that has looked at the post-menopausal woman in Atwood's later fiction (Perrakis 2007 and King 2013). It also complicates Ellen McWilliams's (2009) scholarship on Atwood's *bildungsroman* canon, who uses "maturity" as a critical metaphor to describe Atwood's writing development. I argue that Atwood's canon would benefit from a re-consideration through a spectrum of amaturity.

This chapter offers a reading of Atwood's *Lady Oracle* through a spectrum of amaturity. I begin by defining the female *bildungsroman*, and the adaptation indicated in the weight loss coming of age novel. I then go on to summarize recent developments in intellectual thought regarding fatness, gender and sexuality, drawing upon Judith Butler's gender performativity theory (1990; 1993), and Natalie Boero's (2012) findings on heteronormative weight loss culture. I discuss how fat subjects are abjected through Julia Kristeva's theory of abjection (1982) and the specific relationship this has with notions of maturity. I will then move on to the textual analysis of *Lady Oracle* and Joan's experience as she becomes a gendered object-for-others. Finally, in my conclusion I propose new ways of reading the end of the novel in light of my interpretation.

The *bildungsroman*, although a traditionally masculinist genre (DuPlessis 1985, Labovitz 1986, Fraiman 1993 and Felski 1989), has been reworked by women writers since the 1970s to consider ideas of female youth. According to Rita Felski (1989), the timeframe and place of marriage in the heroine's development and social awakening offers a significant alteration to the form of the *bildungsroman*:

> Marriage, as that mark of narrative closure which exemplifies the merging of individual and social interests, is now explicitly revealed not as the endpoint of female *Bildung*, but as its very antithesis, so that female 'youth'—the period of interior and exterior discovery and development—is located at quite different points within a female social biography. (1989, p. 138)

The female *bildungsroman* reflects in its form a radical critique. Through gender, the coming of age novel expands to incorporate the altered, staggered and delayed "interior and exterior" rites of passage that are otherwise naturalized by masculinist rhetoric as universal. Through weight loss, *Lady Oracle* goes further. An equally gendered experience, Joan's maturation is both delayed and socially unstable until she can emerge as an intelligible gendered subject and engage in the typically passively-enacted gender performances that have been naturalized for women, and excluded unconventional female bodies.

To understand how Joan's experience of maturation is influenced by her weight and social perception, it is important to frame this within contemporary gender scholarship that has looked into the 'doing' of gender and sexuality for fat subjects. Since Susie Orbach's *Fat Is a Feminist Issue* (1978), a study that was published two years after *Lady Oracle*, the relationship between fat and gender has remained an infrequent but significant topic in feminist and fat studies discussions. This is due in part to what feminist scholars such as Sandra Bartky (1990), Susan Bordo (1993), and Naomi Wolf (1990) have labelled a normative cultural shift, in which cultural expectations of femininity no longer focus on what a woman is allowed to do but what a woman is allowed to look like: "Normative femininity is [be]coming more and more centered on woman's body—not its duties and obligations or even its capacity to bear children, but its sexuality, more precisely, its presumed heterosexuality and its appearance" (Bartky 1990, p. 80). Following the legal and economic achievements of second wave feminism in the 1970s and the cultural advances made during the sexual revolution under permissive post-war Western governments, the female body became more focused on its sexuality, its sexual promise, and implicit compulsory heterosexuality.

In her thesis on performativity Judith Butler (1990; 1993) pointed out individual actions through the body could have potentially revolutionary consequences for gender emancipation. Gender, Butler states, is reiterated and stabilized as natural through ritualized performative acts. Through understanding gender as continuously constructed rather than as a stable ontology, Butler offers a way of understanding the 'doing' of gender, exploring new platforms for 'undoing' gender through subversion and resistance. However, criticism of Butler's ideas have frequently appeared from fat and disability scholars who argue a constructivist and discursive approach to bodies does not adequately account for material realities or the agency of the body (Bordo 1993, Colls 2007). Matter, as Rachel Colls (2007) points out, is not as passive as Butler's reading unintentionally supports and fat in particular has bodily agency—fat bodies ripple, spill and move independently. David Mitchell and Sharon Snyder also critique the constructivist arguments of Butler and Sander Gilman as contradictory to a disability studies paradigm, since

> … undergirding their rhetoric of constructed deviancy is that they strategically distance their interest in 'abject communities' from the tangible evidence of physical aberrancy. Subsequently, disabled communities that are defined by virtue of the presence of physical differences will be hard pressed to utilize the same rhetorical tactic. (1997, p. 27)

Studies into gender and fatness also echo Mitchell and Snyder's criticism. Jeannine Gailey (2012) and Samantha Murray (2004) have separately observed how fat women do not find the 'doing' of gender as accessible as slim women, and therefore it is harder to 'undo' gender with the politicized force Butler claims.

Fat subjects, and particularly fat women, find it harder to undo gender because they find themselves excluded from the practice of gender. Natalie Boero in a sociological study of weight loss groups and bariatric surgery patients has found "[n]ot unlike transsexuals learning the appropriate doing of gender as adults, fat people, particularly women, have often been excluded from normative patterns of gendered behavior, interaction, and embodiment" (2012, p. 110). Boero's findings highlight the socialized suppression of gender and sexuality in fat subjects that render this social group less gendered, if not de-gendered. The process of losing weight, then, involves a reassertion of heteronormativity, a process that Boero identifies as "relearning heterosexuality, consuming femininity, and becoming visible" (2012, p. 105). In very real terms, the heteronormative process at the heart of weight loss culture is concerned with easing the psychological stress of passing from the other—the abnormal, the abject—and becoming "human."

Abjection is a psychoanalytical concept developed by Julia Kristeva (1982) that describes the transgression of the body's physical and ontological borders. Kristeva describes the abject as "what disturbs identity, system, order. What does not respect borders, positions, rules" (1982, p. 4). Abject bodies are those that disturb meaning: they leak, spill and give way to the bodies' matter. Elizabeth Grosz points out that Kristeva discusses "three broad categories of abjection—abjection toward food and thus toward bodily incorporation; abjection toward bodily waste, which reaches its extreme in the horror of the corpse; and abjection toward the signs of sexual difference" (1994, p. 193). The fat body through its corporeal fleshiness represents all three of these categories; however, it is the third category I want to focus on. According to Kristeva and Grosz, bodies that do not properly signify a gender are perceived as abject because they transgress the border separating self and other, subject and object; these are dual bodies, both and neither gender, that evoke in the onlooker a breakdown of meaning. Within this logic, a body that is signifying an inappropriate sexuality, say, of someone much older or younger (for instance, an elderly woman dressed up like a pre-pubescent girl) also implicates a similar transgression of the border of "sexual difference."

Having established the history of female *bildungsroman* and ongoing discussions of fatness and sexual abjection, this chapter will now explore how these concepts feed into and are transformed in *Lady Oracle*. The first representation to examine is the abjection of Joan. The abjection of Joan's chubby six year old body is inscribed through its hint at and association with sexuality: "with my jiggly thighs and the bulges of fat where my breasts would later be and my plump upper arms and floppy waist, I must have looked obscene, senile almost, indecent; it must have been like watching a decaying stripper" (p. 46). The layering of fat on Joan's young frame locates pubescent sexual possibilities on Joan's pre-pubescent body where none should be. These bulges of fat create a disquieting shadow, making Joan's body "obscene" and "indecent" for both its current and future potential sexuality. Joan recognizes this herself: "No wonder I fell in love with the nineteenth century; back then, according to the dirty postcards of the time, flesh was a virtue" (p. 46). In reading crude pornographic productions as cultural documents Joan reveals her understanding that societal positivity towards women's bodies is grounded in adult sexuality and male desire. To Joan these soft pornographic materials reveal shifting cultural attitudes towards women's bodies throughout history and the constructedness of her own abject status.

Joan's presentation, like that of a "decaying stripper," is apparently unconvincing in its attempt at performing femininity because it perverts the expectations of the assumed audience: if the aging stripper fails in her attempt to appear 'sexy' Joan also fails in her attempt to achieve its pre-pubescent equivalent, she fails to appear demure and pretty. With a body that spills and ripples out of clothes—uncontainable and unbounded—Joan unknowingly transgresses conceptions of feminine innocence. Victoria Boynton describes the association of Joan's abjected fat child body with sexualized innocence as a "paradox" but a paradox that is the very definition of Kristeva's notion of the abject—it "disgusts while it fascinates" (2002, p. 56). Joan's body is rejected and covered up because it signifies sexuality out of place: like the stripper, she transgresses age norms for signifying sexuality and for the radical public display and performance of a sexualized body. Outside of reproductive time, Joan and the aging stripper are referencing sexual signs that are not, or should not, be accessible to them. The child body and the aged body are typically sexually invisible: in Western cultures, children are expected to emerge as sexual beings in puberty, while women beyond menopausal age are traditionally expected to subdue visual cues of active sexuality, womanliness and sexual availability (for instance, by dressing in muted and conservatively cut clothing). Through age, the sexual display of Joan's child body and her imagined equivalent appear "obscene" precisely because their performance, apparently, thwarts its attended audience: their performance, if offering no pleasure to the viewer, appears for the pleasure of the performer alone. In its self-orientation it presents a radical subversion and a reclaiming of sexual performance.

As Joan reaches high school her othering becomes further interlaced with normative concepts of femininity and sexuality. For the conventionally feminine girls, the novel presents high school as a period of coy aversion to the wanted and unwanted attention of boys, illustrated by Joan's friend Valerie: "She wasn't interested—in her opinion, as I knew, he was a pill—but etiquette dictated that she not be too openly rude to him, as that might get her the reputation of being stuck-up" (97–98). The normative thin girls are careful not to be too available to the boys they like and dismissive of the boys they do not. However, unlike her sexually-desired and sexually-desiring friends, Joan notes how she and other fat girls in her school are excluded from the normative social stratum and projected into and perform up to their own set of 'characters.'

Atwood positions these limiting roles on a spectrum of sexuality. Joan first recalls Monica, the masculine butch, who is "accepted by [the boys], more or less, but as another boy. They didn't seem to think of her as a woman at all" (p. 93). The second is Theresa, a sad and lonely girl, who has the "traditional fat-girl reputation" according to Joan. Theresa is othered as both abject and hypersexual through her supposed sexually availability: "no one knew whether or not the rumors were true, that she would 'do it' under the right circumstances, but everyone believed them" (p. 94). Meanwhile Joan crafts an entirely different role for herself within the heteronormative adolescent culture: playing the "kindly aunt" and "wisewoman" Joan is well-liked by the popular girls and becomes a giving and undemanding friend to her classmates who are engaged in the typical courtship rituals (p. 93).

While discussing their sexual experiences and queries, her friends exclude Joan "out of respect, as one would exclude a nun or a saint" (p. 97). Joan finds herself ushered into a sexual role commonly ascribed to matronly older women who are seen to have moved beyond sexual desire through age: "Though immersed in flesh, I was regarded as being above its desires, which of course was not true" (p. 94). Joan notes how her de-sexualization, or assumed asexuality, is something she acquiesced to through a lack of other available roles: " … for the most part I suppressed my interest in sex as completely as I suppressed my interest in war films. There was no available role for me, so I ignored the whole thing as much as possible" (pp. 96–7). Joan's turning away from war films and sex is a normalized and internalized exclusion (women in representations of the war effort; fat women and men in romance). So deep is her internalized difference that even the few crushes Joan develops are not on the same teen idols as her peers ("Although I pretended to, I didn't really join in my friends' collective passion for male singers" (p. 97)) but a figure on the margins of society and culture, a depiction of the god Mercury "that used to appear on the front of the Toronto telephone directory" (p. 97). Influenced by the escapist romance films she watches with her Aunt, Joan's crushes are presented as fictional, cartoonish and quite literally more myth than man, a pattern of projection that follows Joan into adulthood with her lovers.

In comparison to the tentative courtships of the normative thin girls, the fat girl spectrum of teenage sexuality ranges from deviant hypersexuality of Theresa to the de-gendered, pseudo-homosocial bonding of Monica, and finally, the asexual maturity of Joan. What is notable in the representation of available sex and gender roles for fat girls in *Lady Oracle* is a perceived absence of "girlhood" for the fat teen. Theresa, Monica and Joan are unable to gain access to the local and popular culture of girlhood of their peers—a culture of ritualized coyness, romantic idealism and a dedication to feminine mystique—because in basic terms, Theresa and Monica give away too much, either in reported sexual contact or in giving up heterosexual feminine power for homosocial kinship. Joan attempts to find a middle ground, immersing herself in the culture of her peers, stifling all sense of will and opinion in order to secure a safe space in this girl culture rather than abdicate to a heterosexist boy culture:

> I knew everything about my friends, their hopes, their preferences ... But they guessed nothing about me; I was a sponge, I drank it all in but gave nothing out, despite the temptation to tell everything, all my hatred and jealousy, to reveal myself as the duplicitous monster I knew myself to be. I could just barely stand it. (p. 95)

While initially it seems like Joan has found a preferable role, avoiding social ostracism, Theresa and Monica manage to find some form of social and sexual freedom in their ostracism. In contrast Joan barters for social acceptance with repression and performance.

To compensate for her exclusion from her peer group, Joan spends more time with her Aunt Lou in the cinema, watching sentimental films: "I saw a number of *Adult* pictures long before I was an adult, but no one ever questioned my age" (p. 82). Joan's weight is offered as a reason for her access to these new cultural sites: "fat women are not more noticeable than thin women; they are less noticeable ... To the ushers and the ticket sellers I must've appeared as a huge featureless blur. If I'd robbed a bank no witness would have been able to describe me accurately" (p. 82). She attributes her invisibility as a fat adolescent to her perceived aged maturity and discovers that her weight renders her indeterminately aged: "all fat women look the same, they all look forty-two" (p. 82). Through this unintelligibility Atwood grants the fat body with an ambivalent privilege: the unintelligibility of Joan's fat body results in a temporal shift that disrupts her social landscape by excluding her from adolescent activities, giving her access to more adult ones and a social perception of extremely advanced sexual maturity. To return to Millard's definition of adulthood, Joan's 'passing' as a citizen with "full legal status" is shown to be a hollow victory in comparison to cultural validation by her peers. Adult cultural spaces are not especially rewarded or enriching spaces for Joan because she is still situated on the fringe of society with her Aunt, the divorcee and 'other woman' to a married man.

The conception of the fat subject as out of step with time is not exclusive to fiction. Culturally, fat subjects are perceived to live in a form of conflicting temporality that positions the fat body either accelerating towards death, or on a path towards weight loss and 'reform.'[1] The fat subject in Western culture is never living in the present, but anticipating living sometime in the future. When Joan loses weight, it involves both a gender and temporal realignment and she reflects "it was like being born fully grown at the age of nineteen" (p. 141), an idea that Frances Kuffel explores in the different cultural form of memoir: "I'd never had a manicure ... I hadn't even considered it when I was fat ... Manicures say *I'm adult*" (2004, p. 127). Across different narrative forms, the multi-layered representation of the fat body as on the fringe of normativity, femininity, and sexuality equates to a form of queering of the fat body.

Joan's difference is further reinforced when she does become sexually active: "When sexual frankness became fashionable I read a lot of accounts of other people's first sexual experiences ... None of these were like mine" (p. 96). She locates her first sexual experience as one in which a boy falls to his knees in a street and pushes his head into her stomach:

> What did I do? I was stupefied; I was compassionate; I stroked his hair. My hand smelled of Brylcreem for days ... After a few minutes of this he got up, the knees of his pants dripping wet, and walked away. That was my first sexual experience. I went home and ate my sandwich. (p. 98)

Joan interprets this act as sexual and the language of the scene draws upon distinct sexual symbolism: damp knees, the smell of hair gel on hands, and Joan's eating of a sandwich, in lieu of a cigarette, reference post-coitus imagery. Joan even states she could "picture quite clearly the strained, even agonized expression on his face" as he "performed this grotesque though almost ritual act on a muddy sidewalk" (p. 98). The stomach not usually considered a sexual and sexualized body part, becomes so in this exchange. Joan's representation as on the fringe of normative gender and sexual practice is reinforced through this act of "belly worship" (p. 98). In presenting the stomach as an eroticized body part Atwood highlights the fluidity of sexual desire that can be experienced beyond traditional 'sex organs,' a categorization that excludes alternative experiences of sexual desire that do not hinge on penetrative sex. Significantly, Atwood presents the full, voluminous stomach as a sexualized organ unique to the fat woman, with the fat body as sexual *because* of its size, not *despite* it.

However, Joan's interpretation of this exchange as sexual is underpinned with accommodating subordination. Joan interprets this act, and later ones, as sexual because it involves the invasion of her personal space and the

1 Outside of literature and sociology, medical studies also show how fat adolescents tend to reach puberty faster and age more quickly than their peers. See: Paul B. Kaplowitz. "Link Between Body Fat and the Timing of Puberty" *Pediatrics*, 2008. (121) pp. S208-S217.

metaphorical transformation of her body, if temporarily, as "not her own" by the attentions of the man she encounters: "judging from the way he threw his arms around me as far as they could go, his chemistry textbook lying forgotten on the sod, and dug in his fingers, he might have perceived me as a single enormous breast" (pp. 98–9). Experiencing her body as either invisible or grotesque, Joan considers situations where her body becomes 'shared' with another person as a moment of intense intimacy, even if these situations result in her objectification. In her other two sexual experiences a similar association is reinforced. John the 'Italian or Greek' cook pursues her because she is a good worker and "the shape of a wife already" (p. 101); Rob, her cynical colleague, squeezes Joan's knee after she is shot by an arrow at work, associating her bodily trauma with his own near fatal accident at work. In these experiences Joan's body is *seen* and signifies something different: a giving body. When her body is transformed into a shared space where the boundaries between self and other waver, temporarily, she associates with sexual exchange. With John her body becomes a site of reproductive and economic potentiality; with Rob her injury becomes a reference point for shared pain and self-consolation; and finally, with the boy her body becomes a "giant boob" and a site of entwined sexual and maternal symbolism.

Turning from the othering of the fat body through its association with amaturity, I will now focus on the representation of weight loss as central to Atwood's interrogation of womanhood and her adaptation of the *bildungsroman* form. While scholars of the female *bildungsroman* locate re-birth in marriage, in *Lady Oracle* the moment of re-birth appears through an assertion of the self against the mother through eating and dieting: "The war between myself and my mother was on in earnest; the disputed territory was my body" (p. 69). *Lady Oracle*'s depiction of the mother-daughter relationship falls within the same historical moment as feminist psychoanalysts Susie Orbach (1978) and Nancy Chodorow (1978). Fiona Tolan reads Joan's fluctuating weight as a protest in being made over in the image of her mother. Following one of several attempts by Joan's mother to discipline her appetite and visual expression Joan declares: "I had defeated her: I wouldn't ever let her make me over in her image, thin and beautiful" (2007, p. 88). From this psychoanalytical feminist perspective, Joan's body becomes the semiotic zone over which the daughter and mother assert the self.

Furthermore, Sonia Mycak identifies how all of Joan's textual and sexual experiences relate to her relationship with her mother:

> *Lady Oracle* ends with a resolution of Joan's relationship with her mother, a relationship that has been expressed as a preoccupation with death, a divided sense of self, a number of fractured identities, and a problematic relationship

> with food and with the body. It is a relationship that has been imaged in familial networks, bodily drives, sexual relations and textual practices. (1996, p. 119)

Although Mycak examines Joan's relationship with men in her analysis, ultimately the success of Joan's "struggle for subjectivity" (p. 119) is determined by this final "separation from the maternal" (p. 118). The process of maturity for Joan, then, is originally, and primarily, a renegotiation of the self against the mother through the body.

Lady Oracle's "voyage outward" from "the enclosed realm of the familial home into the social world" (Felski 1989, p. 126, p. 134) that typifies the female *bildungsroman* according to Felski, then, is not the marital home, but the childhood home. Joan receives an opportunity to escape the suffocating familial home through the inheritance left to her by her Aunt Lou that comes with the caveat of Joan losing weight. By slimming to a pre-determined weight Joan gains the financial support and psychological and emotional strength to sever ties with her mother and leave her childhood home. Joan's *bildungsroman* journey begins only when she loses weight and achieves financial independence, finally enabling her to leave her mother. It is significant that Aunt Lou, a figure who might have become Joan's surrogate mother in another genre text is now characterized as too unreliable to supplant Joan's mother—Aunt Lou, Joan reflects, dispensed wise advice that "could have several meanings, when you thought hard about them" (p. 88). Instead Aunt Lou provides the financial incentive for Joan to forge her own way out of her situation through independent self-determination.

Weight loss opens up a new social and sexual terrain for Joan. Once she reaches her goal Joan is plunged into womanhood, an experience brought on by her age and weight loss, and finds herself positively visible as a sexual and social being for the first time:

> It was on these bus trips that I first discovered there was something missing in me. This lack came from having been fat; it was like being without a sense of pain, and pain and fear are protective, up to a point. I'd never developed the usual female fears: fear of intruders, fear of the dark, fear of gasping noises over the phone, fear of bus stops and slowing cars, fear of anyone or anything outside whatever magic circle defines safety. I wasn't whistled at or pinched on elevators, I was never followed down lonely streets. (pp. 139–140)

While the negation of the fat body is a painful and discriminatory process when she is fat, Joan discovers this social invisibility resists another form of oppression, that of heteronormative surveillance. With a new found sexual and social visibility, Joan quickly finds this to be an ambivalent freedom. In comparison to her experience as a fat girl, thin Joan discovers her spatial freedom is more limited. She discovers there are now certain streets and certain times of the day that she has to avoid in order to protect herself in her new visibility:

> … when I shrank to normal size I had none of these fears, and I had to develop them artificially. I had to keep reminding myself: Don't go there alone. Don't go out at night. Eyes front. Don't look, even if it interests you. Don't stop. (p. 140)

Joan acknowledges that she has to 'fake' this knowledge of what is safe and dangerous—to her it is not unconsciously enacted like other women and she has to 'learn' these new spatial rules. Joan's learned spatial awareness is emblematic of 'passing thin' that she experiences through weight loss. While critic Patrick Anderson (2010) has theorized the relationship between visibility, spectatorship and the fasting body in spaces like the prison, the clinic and the gallery, Atwood reveals how the spectacle of thinness is also theatrically enacted on the streets, in the home, and in fact, everywhere.

Weight loss offers Joan a fresh start, and an opportunity to re-write her personal history. Crucially, part of Joan's re-citation as a legible gendered subject involves re-writing her history of abjection. In re-creating her past, weight loss also offers Joan a form of self-creation: Joan in becoming her own author turns body into text. Her desire to self-create reveals a compulsion to further reject the mother—in re-writing the self, she re-writes the mother. For Joan the right beginning is key to the right ending: "You can't change the past, Aunt Lou used to say. Oh, but I wanted to; that was the one thing I really wanted to do. Nostalgia convulsed me" (p. 10). Joan compulsively revises her narrative, recycling characters in a frustrated attempt to arrive at the perfect happy ending. Susan McKinstry observes how "she uses nothing new, but recycles names (Joan Foster, Louisa Delacourt) and incidents (her mother in the triple mirror) in several genres until she is satisfied as an artist with the effect" (1987, p. 67). *Lady Oracle* the novel, "Lady Oracle" the poem, and "Stalked by Love," Joan's final Costume Gothic, are an example of this narrative *déjà vu* as they are essentially the same story cast with the same characters. As *Lady Oracle* draws towards its conclusion Joan struggles to keep her fictional and non-fictional from invading each other: "*Redmond drew back puzzled. 'Who is Arthur?' he said*" (p. 323). In the final fantastical sequence Joan begins to confuse her various romantic entanglements and fiction and reality begin to blur.

The collapsing of Joan's worlds climaxes in an image of her past selves lined up theatrically at the center of Joan's fictional maze in "Stalked by Love":

> Two of them looked a lot like her, with red hair and green eyes and small white teeth. The third was middle-aged, dressed in a strange garment that ended halfway up her calves, with a ratty piece of fur around her neck. The last was

> enormously fat. She was wearing a pair of pink tights and a short pink skirt covered with spangles. (p. 341)

Joan refuses the heterosexist logic of the Costume Gothic genre that would see her narrator fulfilled in a happy union with the hero of the narrative, and his former wife affirmed as her malevolent opposite. Instead Joan is faced with distortions of her past selves (including one who has merged with Redmond's first wife) and romance collapses into gothic. They warn Joan and narrator Lady Redmond (now merged into one) of her imminent peril at the hands of her murderous husband, however, they are also configured as separate and alien to Joan: "She was trapped here with these women" (p. 342). The group of women can be explained as a gothic literalization of what Felski calls "the transference of allegiance," of the heroine, "from a heterosexual relationship to one of intimacy between women" (1989, p. 138). As a communion of ghostly women this episode resists feminist triumphalism and shies from the too-comforting trappings of feminist emancipation narratives that Felski describes. The communion serves as a warning of present peril for Joan instead of offering an optimistic future. However, this uncanny self-communion also has revolutionary possibilities for Joan and presents a "visionary hope of future change" (1989, p. 139). In this fantasy Joan stops running away from her past and faces herself, or selves, which signals Joan's first positive step towards gaining control over her split subjectivity that threatens to consume her. If, as Felski argues, the female communion "involves overcoming the negative value which women have been conditioned to place upon their own sex" (1989, p. 138) in this act Joan overcomes the negative value she has placed on herself for her imperfections, her 'messiness' and lack of coherency.

My reading of the self-communion as one of self-acceptance can be supported in Joan's turn to science fiction writing. To establish my position I will engage with some alternative readings of the final chapter. The novel ends with Joan's discovery by an unknown reporter, who will soon reveal Joan's deception to the world, and his subsequent injury in a physical struggle with Joan. Afterwards Joan nurses the largely indescribable man (indescribable through his apparent featureless ordinariness) and the novel ends with the strong possibility that her identities will be exposed. Frank Davey (1984) makes a compelling argument for Joan's continued entrapment in her Gothic plots through this altercation:

> Her attack with the Cinazo bottle is merely another instance of her fantasizing a man to be a Gothic villain; her decision to stay with and help her victim seems based not on a new sense of self but on the 'nurse' fantasy which patterned the novels of her first lover Paul … (1984, p. 76)

Fiona Tolan (2007) makes a similar case, arguing that Joan's musing, "I guess it will make a pretty weird story, once he's written it" (p. 344) indicates that at the end of the novel Joan has become "trapped in a nightmarish cycle of narrative" (2007, p. 64). The cyclical nature of *Lady Oracle* supports Tolan's reading that the end of the novel is also the beginning as Joan begins to tell her story to the reporter.

However, while the journalist may collapse Joan's story into narrative, she does not relinquish her own status as author. This time Joan resists the sensational draw of gothic romance for the promise of science fiction. In doing so she turns from the past to the future, the unknown and the possible: "The future doesn't appeal to me as much as the past, but I'm sure it's better for you" (p. 345). With a new interest in writing future worlds based on what can be instead of what is, *Lady Oracle* ends where Joan can imagine moving forward as a woman writer, a woman with a divided selfhood and a "reformed" fat subject consumed by her past and potential selves. While not radical, the conclusion of the novel shows an unseen propensity for compromise, self-union and self-forgiveness that previously exacerbated Joan's ontological breakdown.

In situating weight loss as the event that ushered in Joan's burgeoning womanhood Atwood refuses the biological logics of sexual development and the legal signifiers of adulthood. Atwood's emphasis on societal norms as dictating receptions of maturity challenges conceptions of girlhood as either a positive time of shared experience, or a time of self-rejection and an awakening to gender servitude. I argue that girlhood itself cannot be taken for granted in weight loss coming of age narratives like *Lady Oracle* where Joan struggles to be gender cited/sighted in girlhood. Instead of awakening to the restrictions of her gender, Joan instead strives for acceptance within the heteronormative paradigm, an aspiration that leads to a perilously split subjectivity. Fatness, as well as gender and sexuality, appears as an ambiguous but nevertheless powerful transformative experience for Joan's identity.

Through *Lady Oracle*, a watershed text in the weight loss subgenre of the female *bildungsroman*, I have established fatness and weight loss as intimately connected to Joan Foster's experience of girlhood and womanhood, and her suppression of selfhood and sexuality. In examining the appropriation of sexual maturity as a metaphor for weight loss in fiction, I argue that weight loss narratives, while presenting weight loss as formative, exacerbate split subjectivity and fail to return on the promise of happiness and self-satisfaction. In understanding the conceptual frameworks that are used around weight loss, I argue the representation of fatness is also drawn sharply into focus. In looking at a novel that explores the fluidity between states of fatness and thinness, the radical thinking in novels that feature fat characters outside of these paradigms will also come to stand out. Through fat studies criticism and gender and gender theory I have opened up this area of discussion but more needs to be done to uncover the intersections between fatness, sexuality and maturity and the largely uncollected, unknown and diverse fictions where fatness appears plentiful both within and beyond metaphor.

References

Anderson, P. (2010). *So Much Wasted: Hunger: Performance, and the Morbidity of Resistance.* Durham: Duke University Press.

Atwood, M. (1976). *Lady Oracle.* Toronto: McClelland and Stewart.

Bartky, S. L. (1990). *Femininity and Domination: Studies in the Phenomenology of Oppression.* New York: Routledge.

Boero, N. (2012). *Killer Fat. Media, Medicine, and Morals in the American "Obesity Epidemic."* New Brunswick: Rutgers University Press.

Bordo, S. (1993). *Unbearable Weight: Feminism, Western Culture and the Body.* London: University of California Press.

Boynton, V. (2002). The Sex-cited Body in Margaret Atwood. *SCL/ÉLC, 27* (2), 51–70.

Braziel, J. E., and LeBesco, K. (eds). (2001). *Bodies out of Bounds: Fatness and Transgression.* Berkeley and Los Angeles: University of California Press.

Butler, J. (1993). *Bodies That Matter: On the Discursive Limits of "Sex."* New York: Routledge.

Butler, J. (1990). *Gender Trouble: Feminism and the Subversion of Identity.* New York: Routledge.

Chodorow, N. (1978). *The Reproduction of Mothering: Psychoanalysis and the Sociology of Gender.* Berkeley: University of California Press.

Colls, R. (2007). Materialising bodily matter: Intra-action and the embodiment of 'Fat.' *Geoforum*, 38, 353–365.

Crawford, R. (1980). Healthism and the medicalization of everyday life. *International Journal of Health Services: Planning, Administration, Evaluation*, 10 (3), 365–388.

Davey, F. (1984). *Margaret Atwood: A Feminist Poetics.* Vancouver: Talonbooks.

Dawson, C. (1993). *Body of Knowledge.* New York: Algonquin Books of Chapel Hill.

DuPlessis, R. B. (1985). *Writing Beyond the Ending: Narrative Strategies of Twentieth-Century Women Writers.* Bloomington: Indiana University Press.

Ellmann, M. (1993). *The Hunger Artists: Starving, Writing and Imprisonment.* Cambridge: Virago.

Felski, R. (1989). *Beyond Feminist Aesthetics: Feminist Literature and Social Change.* Cambridge, Massachussetts: Harvard University Press.

Fraiman, S. (1993). *Unbecoming Women: British Women Writers and The Novel of Development.* New York: Columbia University Press.

Fuderer, L. S. (1990). *The Female Bildungsroman in English: An Annotated Bibliography of Criticism*. New York: MLA.
Gailey, J. A. (2012). Fat Shame to Fat Pride: Fat Women's Sexual and Dating Experiences. *Fat Studies Journal*, 1 (1), 114–127.
Goodman, W. C. (1995). *The Invisible Woman: Confronting Weight Prejudice in America*. California: Gurze Books.
Grosz, E. (1994). *Volatile Bodies: Toward a Corporeal Feminism*. Bloomington: Indiana University Press.
Hall, G. S. (1904). *Adolescence: Its Psychology and its Relations to Physiology, Anthropology, Sociology, Sex, Crime, Religion, and Education*. New York: Appleton.
Hite, M. (1989). *The Other Side of the Story*. Ithaca and London: Cornell UP.
King, J. (2013). *Discourses of Ageing in Fiction and Feminism: The Invisible Woman*. New York: Palgrave Macmillan.
Kristeva, J. (1982). *Powers of Horror: An Essay on Abjection*. New York: Columbia University Press.
Kuffel, F. (2004). *Passing for Thin: Losing Half My Weight and Finding My Self*. New York: Broadway Books.
Labovitz, E. K. (1986). *The Myth of the Heroine: The Female Bildungsro man in the Twentieth Century: Dorothy Richardson, Simone de Beauvoir, Doris Lessing, Christa Wolf*. New York: Peter Lang.
Lebesco, K. (2004). *Revolting Bodies?: The Struggle to Redefine Fat Identity*. Amherst and Boston: University of Massachusetts Press.
McKinstry, S. J. (1987). Living Literally by the Pen: The Self-Conceived and Self-Deceiving Heroine-Author In Margaret Atwood's *Lady Oracle*. In B. Mendez-Egle., *Margaret Atwood, Reflection and Reality* (pp. 58–70). Edinburgh and Texas: Pan American UP.
McLennan, R. (2009). *Adolescence, America, and Postwar Fiction: Developing Figures*. Basingstoke: Palgrave Macmillan.
McLennan, R. (2013). Cautionary Whales? Adolescence and Genre in Juno and Push. *Mosaic: A Journal for the Interdisciplinary Study of Literature*, 46 (2), 105–121.
McWilliams, E. (2009). *Margaret Atwood and the Female Bildungsroman*. Farnham: Ashgate.
Millard, K. (2007). *Coming of Age in Contemporary American Fiction*. Edinburgh: Edinburgh UP.
Mitchell, D. T., and Snyder, S. (1997). *The Body and Physical Difference: Discourses of Disability*. Ann Arbor: University of Michigan Press.
Mycak, S. (1996). *In Search of the Split Subject: Psychoanalysis, Phenomenology, and the Novels of Margaret Atwood by Sonia Mycak*. Toronto: ECW Press.
Orbach, S. (1978). *Fat is a Feminist Issue*. New York and London: Paddington Press.
Perrakis, P. S. (ed.). (2007). *Adventures of the Spirit: The Older Woman in the Works of Doris Lessing, Margaret Atwood, and Other Contemporary Women Writers*. Columbus: Ohio State University Press.

Ridout, A. (2011). *Contemporary Women Writers Look Back: From Irony to Nostalgia.* London: Continuum.

Rishoi, C. (2003). *From Girl to Woman: American Women's Coming-of-Age Narratives.* New York: State University of New York Press.

Rosowski, S. J. (1988). "Margaret Atwood's Lady Oracle: Fantasy and the Modern Gothic Novel." In J. McCombs., *Critical Essays on Margaret Atwood.* (pp. 197–207). Boston: G. K. Hall.

Tolan, F. (2007). *Margaret Atwood: Feminism and Fiction.* Amsterdam: Rodopi.

Weiner, J. (2001). *Good in Bed.* New York: Washington Square Press.

White, B. A. (1985). *Growing up Female: Adolescent Girlhood in American Fiction.* Westport: Greenwood.

Williams, E. (2009). *Margaret Atwood and the Female Bildungsroman.* Farnham and Burlington: Ashgate.

Wolf, N. (1990). *The Beauty Myth: How Images of Beauty Are Used Against Women.* New York: Random House.

Chapter 13

Flesh Home: The Uncanny Female Architecture of Blake Butler's *EVER*

Laura Ellen Joyce

> Within the psychic architecture that is *EVER*, Blake Butler explores the way bodies swell and contract, going from skin to house and back again. And the way houses too shrink to fit us first like clothing and then like skin and then tighter still. The result is a strange, visionary ontological dismemberment.
>
> (Brian Evenson)[1]

There is a strong relationship between sexuality, flesh, and spatiality in Blake Butler's experimental novella *EVER* (2009). Brian Evenson's argument, stated above, that Butler achieves an "ontological dismemberment," is a useful description of *EVER*, and it is a way in to understanding the Alice in Wonderland weirdness of the way that the unnamed female protagonist fits into her home. She becomes part of the furniture, her teeth and hair become decorations, there are endless, capacious rooms that are full of hauntings, dead mothers and blood; yet the house is so small that she has to crawl through it and often gets devoured by the shrinking walls, or the hungry bath. Her flesh too, is described as endless, filling the entire house; she is "stretched" (Butler, 2009, p. 38), "swelling" (2009, p. 79) and "fat" (2009, p. 10). Her fatness is figured as sexually enticing and yet repellent, her flesh a comfort and a terror. Caroline Narby and Katherine Phelps in their article 'As Big as a House: Representations of the Extremely Fat Woman and the Home' (Narby and Phelps, 2013) refer to Jane Blocker's earlier work on the hybrid "woman-house."

> In her article "Woman-House: Architecture, Gender, and Hybridity in *What's Eating Gilbert Grape?*" Jane Blocker describes how Bonnie Grape becomes a "woman-house," a hybrid figure whose very body is merged with the home. The idea of this kind of "hybridity" between woman and structure, an image of a woman's body either literally or conceptually conflated with the physical structure of a house, is not the province of obscure fantasy, but is an integral aspect of popular representations of the extremely fat woman (Narby and Phelps, 2013, p. 157).

1 From the first edition of Butler, B. (2009) *EVER*, New York: Calamari Press.

The "extremely fat woman" in Blocker, as in Narby and Phelps, is hemmed in and repressed by her integration with the structure of the house. In Butler, the "extremely fat woman" as house is the return of the repressed; she bleeds beyond the borders of structure and exists as radical excess. In *EVER* there is an uncanny geography of fat female flesh; a flesh home that is at once desirable and terrifying. Though I find Evenson's description of the book as achieving an 'ontological dismemberment' a useful one, there seems to be more evidence pointing towards an ontological wholeness—a fusion of flesh and home that is insoluble.

Freud's theory of the uncanny can offer an insight into *EVER*, particularly his arguments on the ambivalent status of the womb. In his essay on the uncanny, Freud discusses 'neurotic men' who feel that there is something uncanny about the female genital organs:

> It often happens that neurotic men declare that they feel there is something uncanny about the female genital organs. This unheimlich place, however, is the entrance to the former Heim [home] of all human beings, to the place where each one of us lived once upon a time and in the beginning. 'Love is home-sickness'; and whenever a man dreams of a place or a country and says to himself, while he is still dreaming: 'this place is familiar to me, I've been here before,' we may interpret the place as being his mother's genitals or her body. (Freud, 2003, p. 15)

There is a clear description of a nostalgia, or home-sickness for youth (in this case extreme, inter-uterine, youth) which is experienced by a man, for the body of a woman, in fact, for time within the womb. This is a way of avoiding finitude, by regressing to the pre-birth period. This is a strategy which is doomed to fail, and which cannot be fully realized. This neurotic ambivalence to the female genitalia describes sexual attraction as a negative, immature experience, which avoids futurity at all costs in a relentless search for the past. This desire to be consumed by the body of the mother (or the mother figure as sexual partner) can be realized as a desire for fat female flesh; a fantasy of flesh as an all-consuming womblike structure.

There is a conflation, in *EVER*, between the homely and the terrifying: The plain, tract housing complex, which is the setting for *EVER*, shows aggressively ordinary, middle American homes, to be places of horror, wonder and awe. The nameless, female protagonist of Butler's *EVER* says: "I found myself inside my sofa. Found I'd squeezed my skin between the crease" (Butler, 2009, p. 70) and "My muscles made a moor" (2009, p. 29).

The ordinariness of the surroundings is seen as a backdrop to extraordinary, supernatural experiences—the sofa becomes a maze; a prison; an extension of the female body. The horror in Butler's work is at once banal and terrifying—there is no specific narrative arc, and no named victim. Butler shows horror to be inherent in the architecture of the novel; what is terrifying is the building itself, part female monster, part haunted house. The protagonist is occasionally dead, she occupies a haunted space where she speaks through her mortal and vivid woundings—where her death should have happened several times, but somehow is always delayed by the magic of the book. Her ambivalent status as between life and death can be related back to Freud's conflation of womb, home and tomb—the feminine monster is seen as such because of her uncanny ability to reproduce, and the way that her flesh becomes the crucible and repository of children. Yet the fat woman is seen as doubly threatening: able to conjure alien subjects from her womb and also aligned to death or the tomb. Narby and Phelps unpick this relationship between home and tomb in the extremely fat woman:

> [T]he extremely fat woman is not only marked for death, but embodies death as a concept, and threatens those around her with annihilation. Her body is a site of radical ambivalence, where both attraction and violent revulsion collide. She is constructed as a physical and emotional burden, a drain on community resources, and a failed woman because she requires "special" care and support instead of maternally bestowing it. Her very physical existence is regarded as antithetical to life, and as such she must be obliterated. She is a dead woman walking. The house is not her sanctuary, but her tomb. (Narby and Phelps, 2013, p. 157)

This radical ambivalence is at the heart of *EVER* and yet it is the protagonist herself who embodies home, womb and tomb; that most uncanny of constellations.

Barbara Creed's extensive work on the 'monstrous feminine' continues this investigation and is a useful text in terms of both the horror genre, and the female uncanny in particular. In her book, *The Monstrous Feminine* (1993), Creed investigates the misogyny inherent in much contemporary horror, and explores representations of the feminine in the psychoanalytic and the symbolic, as well as through direct representation of female characters. Creed describes the womb in horror films as follows: " … The womb is represented in the horror film in at least two main ways: symbolically in terms of intra-uterine settings and literally in relation to the female body. In many films the monster commits her or his dreadful acts in a location which resembles the womb. These intra-uterine settings consist of dark, narrow, winding passages leading to a central room, cellar, or other symbolic place of birth" (Creed, 1993, p. 51). That the monstrous feminine is experienced in the presence of the metaphorical womb is a staple of horror cinema, yet the intimate, probing gaze which is visited upon the metaphorical female body can also be read as a gaze trained on fat female flesh. Narby and Phelps describe this gaze as follows:

> It must be understood that the motivation behind the prying public gaze is much more sinister than stealing a thrilling peek at a monstrous image. The hateful discourse driven by a conflation of fatness and death does not stop at shutting the very fat woman into and merging her with the home; it actively seeks her destruction. (Narby and Phelps, 2013, p. 157)

If the horror house is a womb-like structure, its endlessness and excess can also be viewed as a rendering of the fat, female body. When Butler describes the structure of the house in terms of viscosity, "Deeper down the liquid's thickness ate the glow and scrunched the space to gone" (Butler, 2009, p. 88), there is a strong connection here between the amniotic and the fleshly: just as the liquid continues to fill the space in an excessive, infinite way, so too fatness is figured as a devouring, unstable force which takes up an infinite amount of space. The thick liquid fills the space and blots out the architectural structure; the space once perceived, is now gone. There is an echo of this function in Viedler's *Architectural Uncanny* which describes space as "a devouring force" which "pursues ..., encircles ..., digests ... " (Viedler, 1994, p. 186). Space in Viedler's conception can be seen as combining both the viscosity of fatness and the devouring space of the womb. The monstrous womb, as theorized by Creed, is here invoked as a kind of live burial, which holds a thrill, even as it produces fatal results. To go back, once again to Freud's essay on the uncanny, he also speaks of this thrill of live burial:

> To some people the idea of being buried alive by mistake is the most uncanny thing of all. And yet psycho-analysis has taught us that this terrifying phantasy is only a transformation of another phantasy which had originally nothing terrifying about it at all, but was qualified by a certain lasciviousness—the phantasy, I mean, of intra-uterine existence. (Freud, 2003, p. 17)

The "glow" which has been "eaten" by the liquid thickness, is referred to earlier in *EVER* as part of the body of the narrator: "My body, plump as ever—rung with soft-stitched patterns of grown-out glow. My bag of belly with no baby. My titties stung. My hair knotted full of where I'd been once" (Butler, 2009, p. 38). It is the empty womb, which causes pain to the narrator, and the glow, which she has lost, is subsumed, in the later passage to the womb-like structure of the house. Water is also explicitly related to the womb in a passage at around this section of the book: "I felt an ocean, or something liquid, flushing through the insides of my skin, around my abdomen or womb. A gush or warming throb" (Butler, 2009, p. 33). This proliferation of slippery, watery excess connects the maternal to the fleshly; yet this gush of fluid could also represent the distended, fat abdomen or sexual excretions. The cultural anxiety over the childless woman, considered to be dangerously independent can be seen here as intensified by the image of a woman who has a "bag of belly with no baby"; perhaps the fat woman haunts as a symbol of the ambiguous woman who presents as maternal and reveals her secret; her belly is full and her womb is empty.

It is the confusion of the space, the ambiguity between the womb of the home, the womb of the mother, and the womb of the protagonist, each of which are described as committing violence, or having violence done to them, which aligns this novel to the monstrous feminine of Creed: "Representation of the womb as a place that is familiar and unfamiliar is acted out in the horror film through the presentation of monstrous acts which are only half-glimpsed or initially hidden from sight until revealed in their full horror" (Creed, 1993, p. 51). The links between the wombs of the mother and daughter are one of the ways in which sexual attraction and desire are played out in *EVER*. The necrophiliac relation between the protagonist and her dead, wounded mother, her vanished father, the boys who come to the house to torture her, her masturbatory practices, are all part of the sadomasochistic fantasy narrative which is at the heart of *EVER*.

This sadomasochism is played out through sensual and sexual experiences which relate to both the masturbatory and the gustatory: "The next room was stained with thrumming, beaten awful, seeping up with cruddy flesh, splashed in the seep of acid from certain stomachs" (2009, p. 63) and "I lay gummed up in the grunting, my skin against my skin. My mouth filled with old aromas of my stomach, in my goo" (2009, p. 76). If those last lines speak of masochism there is also a section which reveals the protagonist's sadistic desires. The TV screen, a staple of the American home, is shown in all its uncanniness—it's haunted, consuming, disembodied power shows the viewer more than first appears: "I'd seen on TV as the fifty-yard line became a blister and all those padded men smeared to zero—how quick the broadcast went to blackness and then the blackness went to fuzz and then the fuzz went to an ad for breakfast sausage which I must say looked quite delicious" (Butler, 2009, p. 46). There is an interesting juxtaposition here between the blurred, sparking nature of the spaces between television programmes (the white noise and visual crackle which remains, often colloquially called "snow") and the banality of the sausage advertisement. The word choices serve a dual function in this passage; we recognize the two sets of images as fairly mainstream—one a football game, and the other an advert for breakfast sausage. By interspersing these cultural artefacts—televized national sport and an advertisement for processed foods—with poetic, visual interventions, the reader is forced to analyse and interrogate their relationship with representations which appear to be natural or ordinary. The deep irony of contemporary sports sponsorship by companies such as McDonald's and Coca-Cola is also challenged here and reminds us of what is at stake for toxic food conglomerates in maintaining an ideological link with the health industry whilst contributing to poor nutrition and negative associations with fatness. The fifty yard-line becomes a 'blister"; this connotes both pain and healing—a cushion against worse devastation, yet, also a signifier that damage has happened. The padded men "smear to zero," and there is an unambiguous nod to death here. The repetition of 'blackness' and 'fuzz' to describe the shift in the programmes on the channel, indicates a kind of external supernatural force—a hand controlling the screen. The final bathetic description of the advert for breakfast sausage, is humorous, as it undercuts the darker tone of the passage. It also reminds the reader of the connection between the everyday, the banal and the ghostly.

Butler uses food as a metaphor several times in the novella, and the idea of digestion, peristalsis and defecation are often paired with ideas of home; for example, at one point the protagonist says: "I dreamed there was a door inside my stomach. It was gray and had a curtained window. I could feel the doorbell on my tongue" (Butler, 2009, p. 21). This sometimes nasty pairing is one strategy that Butler uses to conflate the human and the home, and to create a version of the female uncanny which is viewed from a masculine point of view.

In Freud's reading of the female genitals as an *unheimlich* or uncanny space for a man who experiences them, there is a gap which is not addressed—and that is of same sex desire between women. For a woman, desiring another woman, there is likely to be less of an uncanny response, and this is explored in Butler's text. In *EVER*, the figure of the father is seen as distant. However, the relationship between the narrator and her mother is present, and full of anxious desire. The womb is described, sometimes obliquely, as an object which belongs interchangeably to the woman and her mother. Additionally, the home, is also seen as an adjunct to both the woman and her mother. There is an impossibility to this relation, just as there is to the conflation of anatomy and building. In one description, the body of the mother is described as follows: "Her sores were smaller underwater. From above they looked like homes" (Butler, 2009, p. 42). There is abject horror in the description—the sores which rend the body of the mother stretch and shrink under different conditions—the water, a stand-in for the fluid of the womb—relieves the violence and disease suffered by the mother—however, the more striking description—"from above they looked like homes" is unsettling. It combines a reminder that the home is always paired with the rotting female body, and it also shows that the uniformity of the tract houses, if viewed from above, can be considered a blot on the landscape, literal eyesores. The stretching action of the sores reminds the reader of the swelling female body; this swelling is intensified through the lens of the water which distorts and distends.

There are several examples of sexualized exchanges between the narrator and each of her parents, and these can be related back to Kristeva's theory of the abject. Kristeva's book *The Powers of Horror* (Kristeva, 1984) considers the psychoanalytic concept of the abject as that which is cast out of the symbolic order; neither subject nor object the (a)bject is *a-* or outside, beyond, the category of object or subject. For Kristeva the abject relates to filth and decay, corpses and shit; those things which force us to understand the horror of our biological mortality. Kristeva also dramatizes the incestuous sexual desires which occur between child and parent in this category of the abject, or the horror too great to be realized. In *EVER* there are also sexual relations between the narrator and the house itself, and this sexual relation is framed as a narrative of rape, which opens up an investigation into narrative of sadomasochism and coercion.

Early in the novel, when the disoriented reader is still trying to feel their way through the world of *EVER*, there is a section which introduces the district, with its identical, tract houses, which after an unexplained apocalyptic event, are largely empty: "Most of the homes remained undaunted, silent, though one man answered in his flesh bright white and ripped with rashing. I tried to understand" (Butler, 2009, p. 5). This passage introduces the theme of home as sexuality—the homes themselves are given human characteristics—they are "undaunted." The man who answers, has bright white flesh—the expanse of which indicates nakedness, as he is not described as clothed—he is also "ripped with rashing," a violent, visual symbol of blood raised to the surface of his nakedness—the sexual implications are clear. If, as is evidenced in the rest of the text, women are conflated with their homes, then here, the man inside the house, answering the call with his 'rashing' flesh, can be seen as entering into some kind of sexual exchange with the house itself. Soon after this passage, there is the description of what is known as a 'warp' or shift in the atmosphere. The warp can be felt through the medium of the house, and household goods conduct the energy it releases; this energy is described in distinctly sexual terms: "Sometimes there'd be forewarning—a small eruption, more luminescence, an ache or hum of heat in rising steam—though you couldn't recognize the warping til you'd lost a hand or head" (Butler, 2009, p. 8). This rise in pressure, leading to a loss of 'head or hand' can be considered in psychoanalytic terms as a fear of castration, or terror of the monstrous feminine. This is swiftly followed up with a passage I have already mentioned: "I'd seen on TV as the fifty-yard line became a blister and all those padded men smeared to zero—how quick the broadcast went to blackness and then the blackness went to fuzz and then the fuzz went to an ad for breakfast sausage which I must say looked quite delicious" (Butler, 2009, p. 8). This passage bears repeating in this context, as it continues the theme of the sexualized energy which is conducted through ordinary household objects, and it also shows the sadomasochistic desires of the narrator, who conflates the smearing, the zeroing of the athletic men on the screen with the deliciousness of sausage. There is a clear, and humorous, link between the sadistic squashing of these men in their sexual prime, and the devouring of sausage meat—an absurd, yet everyday, marker of the phallic. This tendency toward sexual non-consensuality, is heightened when the protagonist states "I have heard there are men and women who fantasize of rape" (Butler, 2009, p. 17). The erotic devourment described here is a way into thinking about the constellation of fat, food and sex which positions the fat woman as culturally monstrous. The alienating otherness of the gustatory pleasure which the protagonist has in the fantasy of devouring both sausage and footballers dramatizes cultural anxiety over the fat woman and this anxiety is a sadomasochistic one; the fear of being devoured by fat flesh reveals an excitement, a desire. The unusual formation of "I have heard that there are men and women who fantasize of rape" raises questions about normative cultural associations around rape and non-consensuality. In this formation, there are both men and women who fantasize of rape, implicit in this formation is the idea that rape may be enacted by both men and women. By imagining a monstrous female who is capable of enacting violent sexuality, *EVER* presents a desire which is culturally taboo; which remains abject or outside the symbolic order.

Additionally to the sexual relation with the home, the narrator also has a set of fantasies and anxieties around her parents and a strong sexual attraction to the wounded, potentially dead, mother: "All those old nights she'd spread beside me, writhed in reciting, her weird body humped and lumped and ragged—her voice still endless in my head now—a kind of drill or gum or gun" (Butler, 2009, p. 37). Kristeva explicitly formulates abjection in relation to the incestuous parental relationship and her theory helps to explore the way that the protagonist does not relate in any recognized way to her parents, but rather has a psychotic identification to them which is at once intimate and totally detached.

> Essentially different from "uncanniness," more violent, too, abjection is elaborated through a failure to recognise its kin; nothing is familiar, not even the shadow of a memory. I imagine a child who has swallowed up his parents too soon, who frightens himself on that account, "all by himself," and, to save himself, rejects and throws up everything that is given to him—all gifts, all objects. He has, he could have, a sense of the abject. (Kristeva, 1984, pp. 5–6)

In the same way that the child in Kristeva's imagining has "swallowed up his parents too soon," so the narrator of this novel has devoured her own parents and is continually revisiting the cruelties and intimacies of their life together, to try to understand the fright that she feels. Firstly, her relation to her father is elaborated here: "Bled like those days when I was twenty and my whole womb's load would splot out of me at once, and then again in repetition—in repetition—in—in—and. And. Bled like when even younger I cut my finger there in father's shed and he'd take it in his mouth and suck and suck" (Butler, 2009, p. 102). This relation is strongly associated with devouring, eating and consumption, but it is also linked to menstruation, puberty and sex. In this reading menstruation becomes the abject object; it is excluded from the symbolic order through a double form of distancing; once by its destruction through consumption and once by historicizing it to a past time. Yet, the devoured blood returns again and again; it enacts the return of the repressed. The repetition of 'suck' and 'take it in his mouth' implies a kind of comedic phallic inversion, yet it also highlights the sexual relation between the daughter and her father. The father's shed is also symbolic, another temporary and banal space of ordinariness, where an extraordinary, bloody act has taken place. The reference to her womb is another reminder of the hybridity of spatiality and sexuality in *EVER*. The excessive devouring and consumption can be read as both gustatory and sexual; creating a link between the sexual and physical appetites of the protagonist which is an almost stereotypical trope in representations of fat sexuality.

The description of the relation between the narrator and her mother is more explicit: "In certain spots I heard a humming, some long, slow strum sung through the floor. At times it mimicked mother's tumour babble: nights I'd wake inside the house inside her howl, or humping hard against a bare wall, leaving wet imprints on the plaster" (Butler, 2009, p. 6). There is a pleasurable sensuality inherent in the vibrations which the narrator both feels and hears through the floor. When she wakes 'inside the house inside her howl," there is a synaesthesic quality to the experience. The howl of the mother is animalistic, and it is also a sexual sound—the ways in which these sounds are inescapable, and thrum through the narrator's body, and through the house, indicate that there is something of the primal scene here,[2] that is, the compulsion and repulsion which the child feels towards seeing and hearing her parent(s) in ecstasy, read alternately as horror. By using the phrase "humping hard against a bare wall, leaving wet imprints on the plaster," there is, again, a link between sexuality and spatiality—the clear overtones of fucking are aligned to the materials of the house.

The house, in *EVER*, always returns. It is the repressed which haunts. The house is typical, ordinary and banal, as well as being the site for transcendental horror. In this way, it makes a perfect crime scene. Edward Bond's description of

2 The primal scene according to Freud is the child's first sighting of a sexual act, most often between their parents or parental figure which leads to trauma. See Freud, 1991, pp. 524–525. According to Ned Lukacher "The primal scene has conventionally been theorised as the observation by the child of the parental couple having intercourse; as, the child's witnessing of a sexual act that subsequently plays a traumatic role in his or her psychosexual life" (Lukacher, 1986: 24).

the psychotic crime scene, in his book on Lacan and crime scene photography, *Lacan at the Scene*, is useful in understanding the nature of the house in *EVER* as a crime scene. Bond's theory is that the psychotic crime scene contains a chaotic jumble of the homely and the obscene:

> Elements drawn from the familiar appear to be blurring and combining, their ordinary domestic contexts jettisoned. A packet of Coleman's Instant mashed Potato can be seen next to some worn lady's stockings. Next to this is a large piece of polythene and other textile garments and what looks like underwear discarded on a large pile of unprotected LP records (fragile objects, designed to be carefully returned to their sleeves), a torn book cover, a broken lampshade, fragments of crockery, a lone hair curler. A wider view of the scene—photograph 4.2—reveals a saucepan inexplicably placed on a bedroom cabinet, waste receptacles overturned or unused. In photograph 4.3, a suitcase is depicted with a large hole in it, its contents accessed unconventionally. (Bond, 2012, p. 95)

In *EVER*, there is a close relationship to this psychotic crime scene. The narrator has no grasp on the space of her surroundings and chaos reigns. Objects proliferate and transform, people shift into inanimate objects and shift back again. The narrator says: "In the room now there were several of me standing. There was me and me and me. So many kinds I could not remember, slabs of skin I'd long abandoned" (Butler, 2009, p. 68), and later "All my other versions—I couldn't count them—some were so ugly—they swarmed around—standing, squatting, hung from the ceiling, eating dinner, spinning, touched—I could not look at most of them directly. One of me began to speak" (Butler, 2009, p. 69). This proliferation of selves, is presented as homely—they do simple, everyday things like eating dinner, but they also become similar to furnishings or light fixtures, they "[hang] from the ceiling." In this way the house becomes chaotic, and the mundane tasks of living in a house become tinged with lunacy and terror.

This kind of chaotic background becomes part of every action the narrator takes in the house. The very act of going to bed, to sleep, is charged with violence and pain:

> When I slept with cotton wool in my ear holes (which also helped conceal the roof's in-caving creak, the gunfire and the shouting), the blood would gush up from my nostrils or an older bruise, even those considered healed. Or from my vagina (even in off-times). Or my knuckles or my mouth. Some days I'd wake to find the pillow sopping, chock full and black around the edges. (Butler, 2009, p. 23)

The violence is presented as being omnipresent. The sounds represent the human (shouting), the homely (the roof), and the murderous (the gun)—all of which are essential elements of any domestic crime scene. Bond posited, in his chapter on psychotic crime scenes: "The dysfunctional locale is also a lawless space, a space where generally accepted rules do not apply, and transgression reigns" (Bond, 2012, p. 65). In *EVER*, it would seem that the opposite were true, that in fact the dysfunctional locale that Butler has created is not a lawless space, but that in fact perversion, psychosis and transmutations are the laws which hold the space together—it is the very dysfunctionality which allows the inhabitants of this house to exist. Those who have been described as lost, as from a distant past, are those whose behaviour is not psychotic—in the world of *EVER*, the fantastic, and the impossible, are the only modes of existence.

The house in *EVER* veers between being so tiny that the protagonist leaves smears of flesh and scrapes of bone along its plaster wall—"I pressed my teeth against my teeth. The keyhole saw me writhing" (Butler, 2009, p. 29)—and so endless that it contains hundreds of impossible rooms. Both versions of the house remind the reader of the fatness of the protagonist. As she scrapes her body through the rooms we can feel her swelling to fit the space. Because she has already been conflated entirely with the house we see her body presenting as endlessly as the rooms described. The sheer repetitious onslaught of the descriptions of the rooms remind us of the infinite nature of her body: "The next room was lined with shelves so high I could not see. Some soft choir overhead. Stink of paper rot. I had on a dress that had burned once in a fire" (Butler, 2009, p. 67). This room is infinite; there are shelves which go on forever and which are out of reach. "Some soft choir overhead" conjures images of angels, religiosity and beauty and these soft, angelic, insubstantial figures are weighed against the carnal heft of the protagonist who is fixed firmly in the abject world of rot and decay. Her paper dress which has been burned in a fire connotes decay, death and sacrifice but it also creates an image of partial nakedness and uncovered flesh. By pitting the fleshly protagonist against her ghostly counterparts a central fictional binary is dramatized. Narby and Phelps in their article "As Big as a House: Representations of the Extremely Fat Woman and the Home" state that:

> The prevailing understanding of extreme fatness, even outside of the fictional examples we have analyzed here, is that it kills people. Fat itself becomes an agent of death, and the extremely fat person is marked for death. This signification is reflected in the medical term "morbid obesity," and fat activists who might be considered "morbidly obese" by the medical establishment sometimes refer to themselves as "death fats." Cultural fear of fat and fatness represents, at least in part, the fear of annihilation. This fear sustains a commercial industry dedicated to selling slenderness, which has come to connote "health" and life.

The protagonist is aligned to the abject in this room as she wears her dress of rot but she is also aligned to the "death fats" and she exists at a great distance from the slender angels above.

Another of the room descriptions which has relevance here, is as follows: "the next room was every person and their auras and their shit. *I almost stayed forever in this room*" (Butler, 2009, p. 61). This is an interesting revelation—there is a playfulness between interiority and exteriority here. The room is excessive, it contains everything and also it contains itself. If the room contains every person, and their aura and their shit—we are seeing another abject/sublime marriage—shit belongs quite explicitly to the diseased and ugly world of the abject—along with corpses and refuse. Auras belong to the sublime. However, there is an inherent paradox—how can the room contain every person, and yet the narrator is free to walk in and out of it? If fat is figured as excessive, then so is sexuality and the sexualized fat woman belongs in these rooms where she exists at a place of excess beyond the real. Alain Badiou in his talk "Infinity and Set Theory: How To Begin With The Void"[3] argued that when we conceive of the infinite we must consider ideas beyond human consciousness and experience:

> The infinite says something by itself. So we can begin with the infinite but because the infinite has said something to us. So there is something external, you see, when we begin by the infinite, something which is not the pure beginning but the beginning with something else, something which is outside, something finally transcendent. And it is why in this conception we must have something like a revelation and not pure knowledge. There is a revelation. Something has been said, something has been written outside the beginning itself, the beginning of human being as such. And we return to this problem after when we have the first concept of the infinite.

This trickery with the possible and impossible is a central tenet of the novel, and is what contributes to Brian Evenson's assertion that the book presents an "ontological dismemberment." However, rather than ontological dismemberment, I would argue that, in fact, this novel presents us with a fusion of flesh and home, and with an ontological insolubility.

The very end of the book returns to these ideas of the infinite with a description of an endless balloon, a description which draws comparisons with Donald Barthelme's[4] short story "The Balloon," which describes a balloon which covers the entirety of New York:

---

3 Delivered to the European Graduate School in 2011.

4 Barthelme was an experimental short fiction writer whose work was influential on a generation of later writers. He lived between 1931—1989.

> The big balloon sullied the otherwise clear and radiant Manhattan sky. That is, the balloon was, in each man's view, an imposture, something inferior to the sky that had formerly been there, something interposed between the people and their "sky." But in fact it was January, the sky was dark and ugly; it was not a sky you could look up into, lying on your back in the street, with pleasure, unless pleasure, for you, proceeded from having been threatened, from having been misused. And to the underside of the balloon was a pleasure to look up into, we had seen to that, muted grays and browns for the most part, contrasted with walnut and soft, forgotten yellows. And so, while this man was thinking sullied, still there was an admixture of pleasurable cognition in his thinking, struggling with the original perception. (Barthelme, 2005, p. 116)

It is worth bearing in mind that Butler himself, on the blog *HTML Giant*, which he curates, offered this piece of advice to contemporary writers, perhaps also to himself: "you are writing in a period more than twenty years after the death of Donald Barthelme. Act like it" (Butler, 2010). However, this piece of advice can also be considered to be an affectionate one, acknowledging the debt to Barthelme in this work:

> Pressed in the corner, through the window, I saw the balloon stretched and writhing over all. It'd wrapped around the neighbour's roof and porch—it'd wrapped around the children in the yard—if there were children out there any longer—it'd wrapped around the sideways trees and breeze and sky tines and the plasticine arch where we'd erupted and been stitched. What other things it'd wrapped I could somehow name and not quite name. The balloon, bright pinked and endless, pressed to the divots of my nose. (Butler, 2009, p. 75)

This total immersion in the plasticity of the balloon, it's endlessness, feels progressive—the pink of the balloon, the childlike narrative of play, is a bright spot in the otherwise gloomy world. The pink endlessness of the balloon also calls to mind a return to the womb.

The man-made materials which the housing is built from, and which the objects within the houses are made from, are used as here as political building blocks. The cheapness of the materials reflects the social context of those living in these houses; the MDF and polyresins, the nylons and polyesters are plastic in more ways than one. Plasticity here can be figured as positive—progressive as well as toxic. Plasticity can be figured through queerness and alterity—through what is considered to be refuse and waste. What is excess to requirements is also excessive in a political sense—by reading these locations as marginal, and the inhabitants as outside the mainstream—there is the potential to challenge and transgress normative ideologies. There is a sense of redemptive necrophilia, a connection to the past through ephemera and decay. The endless nature of the balloon, the pinkness, the fatness, the swelling and the stretch speak of an alterity which allows a range of queer sexualities and modes of embodiment, at the same time as a disposable, finite object is invoked. This movement between the finite and the endless creates an ontological wholeness; an insoluble fusion between object and world.

References

Badiou, A. "Infinity and Set-Theory: How to Begin with the Void" (2011) at http://www.egs.edu/faculty/alain-badiou/articles/infinity-and-set-theory/.

Barthelme, D., Gates, D. (2005) *Sixty Stories*, London: Penguin Classics.

Blocker, J. (1996) "Woman-House: Architecture, Gender, and Hybridity in *What's Eating Gilbert Grape*?" in *Camera Obscura* 39 (13) pp. 126–150.

Bond, H. (2012) *Lacan at the Scene*, London: MIT Press.

Butler, B. (2009) *EVER*, New York: Calamari Press.

Butler, B. (2010) The Dead Father is Dead. *HTMLGiant.*

Creed, B. (1993). *The Monstrous-Feminine: Film, Feminism, Psychoanalysis*, London: Routledge.

Freud, S. (2003) *The Uncanny*, London: Penguin Classics.

Kristeva, J. (1984) *Powers of Horror: An Essay on Abjection*, Columbia: Columbia University Press.

Lukacher, N. (1986) *Primal Scenes: Literature, Philosophy, Psychoanalysis*, New York: Cornell University Press.

Narby, C. and K. Phelps (2013) "As Big as a House: Representations of the Extremely Fat Woman and the Home" in *Fat Studies* 2 (2) pp. 147–159.

Vidler, A. (1994) *The Architectural Uncanny: Essays in the Modern Unhomely*, Cambridge: MIT Press.

Creative Interlude

Chapter 14
Coming Out Fat

Kimberly Dark

The two of them stood in the lobby, waiting to say hello after the show was over. They were quite a buddy-duo—one fast-talking, big-smiling and full of compliments. The other, quiet, arms folded across chest, an appreciative smile across her lips. The bolder of the two started talking first.

"That was a great show! And ohmigod, you're totally sexy. I could've looked at you for hours. In fact, I'd like to look at you for a few more hours." The quiet friend nodded with a vaguely flirtatious smirk. The garrulous one continued. "So, what do you need? You need a ride? Someone to buy you drinks? You don't know anyone in this town do you? You're just passing through doing a show, so you're gonna go out with us, right?" She looked at her friend, and back at me. "You're so totally going to go out with us!" The friend added, "It'd be great if you'd like to join us for a drink. I loved the show."

It was a pleasure to meet them, watch them and listen to their foolishness. They'd set up the scene. I was the traveling performer and I'd done my job telling stories about love and life and romance. They were the dandies with drink money. I was hot and they were full of appreciation. The story only had to unfold …

I met the quiet one for lunch a few days later and yes, we became lovers.

This is how it starts. Something pleasurable is set in motion. I do like to be admired, to be seen as beautiful and smart and funny. Who doesn't? She was hot too. And smart and funny. The whole narrative was set in motion from the first meeting.

I've been "the first" for quite a few lovers. They're thin and I'm fat and that's new to them. Mostly we don't talk about it. It's a taboo topic in modern culture. Fat is the antithesis of hot, of smart. Okay, fat can be funny, but that's not sexy. We don't go there. Besides, one tries to be gentle with a new lover's feelings, so I always wonder, when is it appropriate for me to "come out" as fat?

There are so many small considerations in a new dalliance—when do you share intimate things about yourself that might cause a new lover to see you differently? Once you get past the one night stand, you have to find the right moment to let someone know your Dad left when you were five, or your uncle molested you or you drink wine pretty much every night or you once became violent with your ex and then, wow, regretted that, no, really, never doing that kind of stuff again. Never.

When do you come out about picking your nose, wearing a wig because you're partially bald or having the ugliest feet most people have ever seen? Seriously, there are things that might make a person question how lovable you are. Is that going too far? There are experiences and appearances that might not make you seem like an attractive mate. And hey, no one likes to be written off by someone they really like. We want to be flattering to the people we care for, and let's face it, we want them to hold up their end of the bargain and be the kind of people we're happy to introduce to our friends.

So, when do I come out about being fat?

What may seem obvious to anyone looking at me must be made to disappear as if through magic, if I'm also to be thought beautiful, sexy, hot and desirable. And so if fat is to be discussed at all, it must become visible again. Who makes it visible? And when?

Beauty Privilege

It's not like we're creating a fiction. I *am* beautiful and it's in my best interest to be seen that way. Loads of people are beautiful, or they can put on the pretty—wear and do and act in ways that invoke beauty. People rarely pause to think about beauty privilege in Western culture. I often say it all at once: tall-pretty-people-privilege. When one really takes stock, it is so amazingly real.

Women should be about 5'7," men should be about 6'2." We should all be slender, with fairly symmetrical facial features, pale skin and flowing hair. We don't like to admit it; we like the idea that people should be valued for their talent and verve, their beautiful hearts. And this is hogwash in every quick moment and in most extended interactions too. I know about tall, pretty people privilege because I have experienced the rewards. Sometimes a person I don't even know—let's say, a clerk at the post office—looks up to see me and seems mesmerized by the light in my eyes, the movement of my full lips (make-up helps accentuate these features for sure) and the subtle way I emanate sensuality. And suddenly, that person wants to be helpful. It's no wonder women learn how to enhance this response through micro-flirtation, through make-up and clothing that draw attention to the features that create positive outcomes. But here's what's interesting—most people with privilege come to see it as normal—warranted even. They deserve to be treated with that kind of attentiveness and courtesy. They may not even know that less attractive people don't receive the same treatment.

I do know what it's like to be seen as unattractive—because I'm also fat. And nothing cancels out female beauty as quickly as being fat. For many onlookers, fat is actually proof of failure and poor moral character, in addition to causing ugliness. For some, a fat person cannot be considered attractive, no way. The two categories: fat and pretty—are mutually exclusive.

So, I have come to understand the way beauty privilege works because I have been fat and beautiful most of my life. (For short periods, I've been more slender too and indeed, one can get accustomed to the reliability of beauty privilege very quickly.) This is part of what I've learned: beauty really is in the eye of the beholder, and the expectations are cultural. Some people look at me and see a pretty woman. Others look at me and see a fat lady. Both are possible. Both are cultural. And depending on what they see, they treat me very differently indeed. If that same postal worker looks up and sees a fat lady, rather than a pretty one, there is no pleasured, mesmerized look. I am to be moved through the line as quickly as possible. That person will barely have the time to listen to my request. I'm just another annoying fixture in another tedious day. That's what lack of beauty privilege looks like. Sure, there are variations, but that is the overall effect.

So, back to sex. Of course it happens that slender people who have never considered fat people attractive sometimes find me attractive. And I have other charms too—let me not recount them here. Suffice to say that often enough, people think I'm hot and I think they're hot and we start carrying on a hot little number—I'm sure it happens this way for others too.

And sometimes, I'm the first fat lover in the life of a slender person who had never considered that fat people could even be attractive—and so that person's going through some stuff inside. Or alternatively, maybe I'm not the first, and that person has been attracted to fat folks before, but never got over the shame of prolonged or public involvement with someone that many consider ugly and profoundly flawed. That person's also going through some things when we become lovers too because I'm not into being ignored. I'm into be adored. And turning down the dial on MY sexy, vibrant entitlement is not on the agenda.

But seriously, why would a fat person have to "come out" as fat? Isn't fat obvious?

Freedom and Ease

I'll let you in on something you may not know: there are two worlds out there with regard to how people feel about fat. In one world—the one that controls most of the media and sells most of the products, the one that runs the politics and the public works—fat is a travesty. The very word is a terrible insult from which you protect your friends and lovers.

In another world, increasing numbers of people of all body types live happily and healthily and with minimal regard for beauty tyranny. They work and walk and swim and fuck and dance and sleep and get sick and well and love and die without organizing their lives around their hatred or suspicion or judgment of their bodies. Well, they practice living that way at least, because the other world is tough to ignore.

In that second world, fat is just a description, like tall or blonde or deaf. It's not inherently a problem and it's certainly not inherently ugly or unlovable. I live mostly in that second world, but I'm super-aware of how that world is encased in the other. And because of how privilege is invisible to those who have it, it's kind of rare for thin people to participate in the world where fat is just a thing, rather than being a terrible thing.

And it's really too bad that there aren't more thin people in my world, because plenty of them hate their bodies too. In fact, most self-confident fat women have, on occasion, met thin women who are angry with them for living vibrant, relaxed lives when they struggle everyday with unworthiness and body hatred. Sad but true, some body-haters just can't be happy for the rest of us. Sexy fat women are doing a public service by demonstrating another way of living and loving ourselves. We're not easy to ignore and we're not always appreciated for our verve by those who most need help. My thin friends sometimes struggle more with body acceptance than I, and I have compassion for that struggle. My own body-love isn't always easy. It's a conscious choice. I know how making that choice frees me and yet, as my body ages and changes, I have to make the choice again. Most of the time it really works.

I caught my thin lover once, watching me with scrutiny as I moved, nude, around our hotel room packing up a suitcase. When I asked what was on her mind, she said she kept trying to find the lie in my self-acceptance. She kept looking for the truth of my body hatred, but couldn't find it. She was astonished that my comfort seemed real.

Protecting Our Loved Ones

I've been fat and beautiful, living and practicing as I do for long enough that I know there's a lot of potential complexity in how my lover experiences me. Indeed, I'm always re-experiencing myself through them. Body love in a culture of constant assault is sketchy and I have managed it differently at various times in my life. I wonder now if my youthful tendency to be attracted to thin people reflects a desire to distance from oppression. Perhaps it was an internalized oppression wherein people who look like me are not attractive. I have lived in the different worlds myself and I know what it's like to manage un-nameable feelings.

Early in a romance, we're hyper-aware, often quite sensitive to joy and pleasure, the desire for everything to go well. We manage our own feelings and some of the lover's perceptions as well. There's a potential for invoking the pain of body hatred, the shame of beauty failure in anyone. So, when do I talk about being fat?

We have already decided that I'm hot enough that the fat can be ignored, so why re-conjure it? If I can tell that my lover is participating in that lie, it's probably because she wants to. Sometimes I even want to protect my lover from having a fat girlfriend, and so there's a double lie. At least I'm aware of the lie—but she might not be. Wow is this complicated! It's not uncommon in our culture to lie for comfort—and to protect the comfort of loved ones. Once we start talking about fat, we're opening the whole culture for critique and reality could just cave in. We lie all the time! Some people have an easier time discussing the experience of being fat than others. And being fat does not automatically give one an ability to discuss fat. That's part of why couples can often maintain a pact of not discussing it for years.

We're really comfortable with lying to protect one another's frailties. Especially, we lie to people we love. Everyone recognizes this classic exchange: "Honey, does this dress make me look fat?" "No darling, you never look fat." Well, sometimes Darling *is* fat. Sometimes Honey is not just avoiding conflict. Honey is maintaining the comfort of illusion. Everywhere we have rigid standards around gender and respectable behavior; we lie in order to uphold them. There's no other way. Why go tearing apart the very fabric of our cultural illusions when we really want an exciting romance, a little roll in the hay? Just let the passion unfold as passion does. We're into each other—probably for a number of subtle and overt reasons—and we both feel hot for each other. We feel hot, as lovers do, both as the object of another's lust and as the person feeling the turn-on. That's the ideal, right? Don't mess with it. Just flirt and canoodle and eventually, we're getting it on; we're in bed and it's all going well and …

Why mess it up by talking about something that makes people uncomfortable? Making someone overtly uncomfortable is not the road to mutual understanding. And that's really what I want—a lover who understands and respects my experiences. I hope to offer respect and understanding too; after all, intimately exploring different experiences is one of the things that makes a love affair interesting. Go too far with the "diversity" however, and one becomes unrelatable—too different. We constantly negotiate interpersonal comfort.

It's possible to wait too long to discuss fat—to protect each other too much. I had a whole relationship, and engagement with someone once and we'd never said the word. We had talked around it, but for my lover, I was only allowed to be sexy. I was only allowed to be hot, beautiful, smart and fun. I felt I had to protect her from some of my painful and enlightening and funny and bold and triumphant experiences and no matter how well everything else was going, that could get lonely.

When Fat is Not a Problem

But really, flattering clothing aside (literally), why would I need to come out as fat if someone's seen me naked?

Oddly, that's exactly when fat-as-a-problem becomes least noticeable. When we're two people naked in bed there is no side-by-side comparison with smaller women, there are no chairs to fit into, narrow aisles to negotiate. There's no one looking at me and at my partner with the eyes of fat-hatred and wondering why on earth, he or she is with someone like me. Fat-as-a-problem is largely social. When we're in bed, generally things are going really well. The truth is that a wide range of bodies fit together nicely and where there's lust, there's a way. Some body-haters fixate on how difficult it would be to navigate sex with bodies of different sizes, but that's foolishness. They focus on fat people. No one ever wonders how the petite prom queen and the giant muscled football player could possibly get it on even though they are radically different in height or weight. The concern over some bodies being "too big" for sex is nothing but fat hatred looking for expression.

I used to be one of those people who didn't discuss fat easily. In my youth, I hoped to avoid the conversation all together. When I'm the first fat lover for a thin beau, there are moments when "working it through" becomes visible. Back in my early twenties, I remember noting hesitation in my lover's touch as he moved his hand across my belly. I saw an almost puzzled look on his face, and when I asked if something was wrong, he was honest. I wished I hadn't asked, because wow, of course those moments are vulnerable for me too. I didn't want to know, in that moment, that he was "a little freaked out" and "not sure how he should feel about my belly." I remember feeling sadness, and just wanting the silence that comes with the pact of beauty and attraction.

Years later, in my thirties, I felt anger when a thin lover—for whom I was the first—told me over coffee that she wasn't sure what she thought about being with someone "my size." She seemed baffled—and oh-so-entitled to explain it all to me. She found me really hot, even though I was totally big. "I mean, it's like your sexiness erases you being overweight, but then sometimes I look at you and think, wow, I don't know. You know?" I did know, and still I couldn't fathom her audacity! She added, "My friends totally know how much I'm into you, so they suggested kidnapping you for a few weeks and feeding you celery sticks, so, you know, it's not that I'm not TOTALLY hot for you … "

She experienced my restraint, or she'd have been wearing that coffee we were drinking. Instead, I told her she needed to work through her bullshit discrimination on her own—it wasn't my job to enlighten her AND have sex with her. And furthermore, I am NOT "overweight." This IS my weight. I raged for a bit and stormed off, but in the end, her honesty held promise and we had further discussion and further hot sex. Even now, in my forties with a whole lot of body acceptance activism behind me, intimacy is still vulnerable. I still want to feel lovable, beautiful, adored. I still value honesty and understanding who we are both privately and publicly.

Identity Management

So, when do we talk about—forgive the irresistible pun—the elephant in the room? And what is the elephant?

The real problem is not so much that I'm fat as that I carry a stigmatized identity, and association will stigmatize my lover too. There's no getting around it. Sure, there are disclaimers people can make to salvage some respectable social identity—some fat people talk about being on a diet, or about how thin they used to be, or about how it was the pregnancy or the injury or the illness that made them that way. Some fat people and their pseudo-defenders will highlight their super-fitness or super-fashion sense in a quest to shed some stigma, but ultimately, we navigate a fat hating culture. And some of us are fat. The problem is not what bodies do in bed. That works brilliantly—always has and always will—as long as we can let lust be the guide.

This IS what we need to talk about: what does it mean to live with oppression? What does it mean to fetishise thinness (to be so attached to a certain attribute that without it, no turn-on can occur)? What does it mean that we allow privilege and oppression to occur in our culture and to let it remain so profoundly invisible, we'll even collude with one another to reject reality?

And when we start asking these questions, more emerge. In what other ways do we subvert "the obvious" in order to not *need to* restructure social privilege? Does coming out as "fat" in a thin-privilege culture seem a little like coming out as "black" in a white-privilege culture for example? Or coming out as disabled? As long as you don't talk about it, as long as you have other laudable identities to offer, the stigmatized traits might go unnoticed. (Try this: have a read through this chapter again when you're done—substituting black for fat, white for thin—and notice the places where this works with race too.)

These are big questions without easy answers, and once you've come to a place in your life where you start to discuss them, it's tough to go back to mindlessly cooing over each other's perfections. The desire for honesty, peace and liberation become like a song you just can't get out of your head. We begin to notice how bodies exist in culture—and in intimate moments too. And that's why at some point I definitely bring it up—unless my lover brings it up first.

My most recent lover is a thin person and I was her first fat fling. We'd been rolling happily in the hay for a few days when I asked—with very little gravity—"hey, have you ever been lovers with someone as fat as me?"

She said, "No."

And I replied "How's that going for you?"

She smiled, both of us naked in bed, she said lasciviously, "It's going pretty well." Then she added, "but hey, I could ask you the same question. Have you ever been lovers with someone as thin as me?" she caressed her lean flank, bony hip. "I'm a little skinnier than usual these days." She said, looking down at her own body for a moment.

I gave her the once-over, really taking in her thinness. "Maybe not," I shrugged. "It's all going really well from here too," I added.

We kissed. And suddenly, neither of us had further interest in the conversation …

Index